## PRAISE FOR *THE PAIN PROJECT*

"A beautiful, humane, thoughtful inquiry into the challenge of living with chronic pain ... it takes on a daunting topic with heart and humor and determination. It's wonderful."
**SUSAN ORLEAN**, author of *The Orchid Thief* and *The Library Book*

"An extraordinary book, raw, honest, immediate, literate, and astonishingly readable ... an inspiring example of how to deal with the challenges of life itself."
**CAROL SHABEN**, author of *Into the Abyss*

"Dearly intimate and heartbreakingly universal ... an unforgettable inquiry into the deeper meaning of pain."
**MICHAEL HARRIS**, author of *The End of Absence*

"A story of endurance in the face of formidable odds—and a story of enduring love. If you live with pain, or care for someone who does, *The Pain Project* is necessary reading."
**SUSAN OLDING**, author of *Pathologies*

"A medicine cabinet of wonders ... stacked with loving wisdom, revelatory research, and all the right questions." **AVI LEWIS**, filmmaker and activist

"Stanley bravely tells the intimate story of a relationship any reader would envy despite its pain."
**BONNIE SHERR KLEIN**, OC, author and disability activist

"A road map through the very human experience of pain." **KENNETH R. ROSEN**, author of *Troubled*

"Utterly fascinating and inspiring."
**ANDREAS SCHROEDER**, author of *Renovating Heaven*

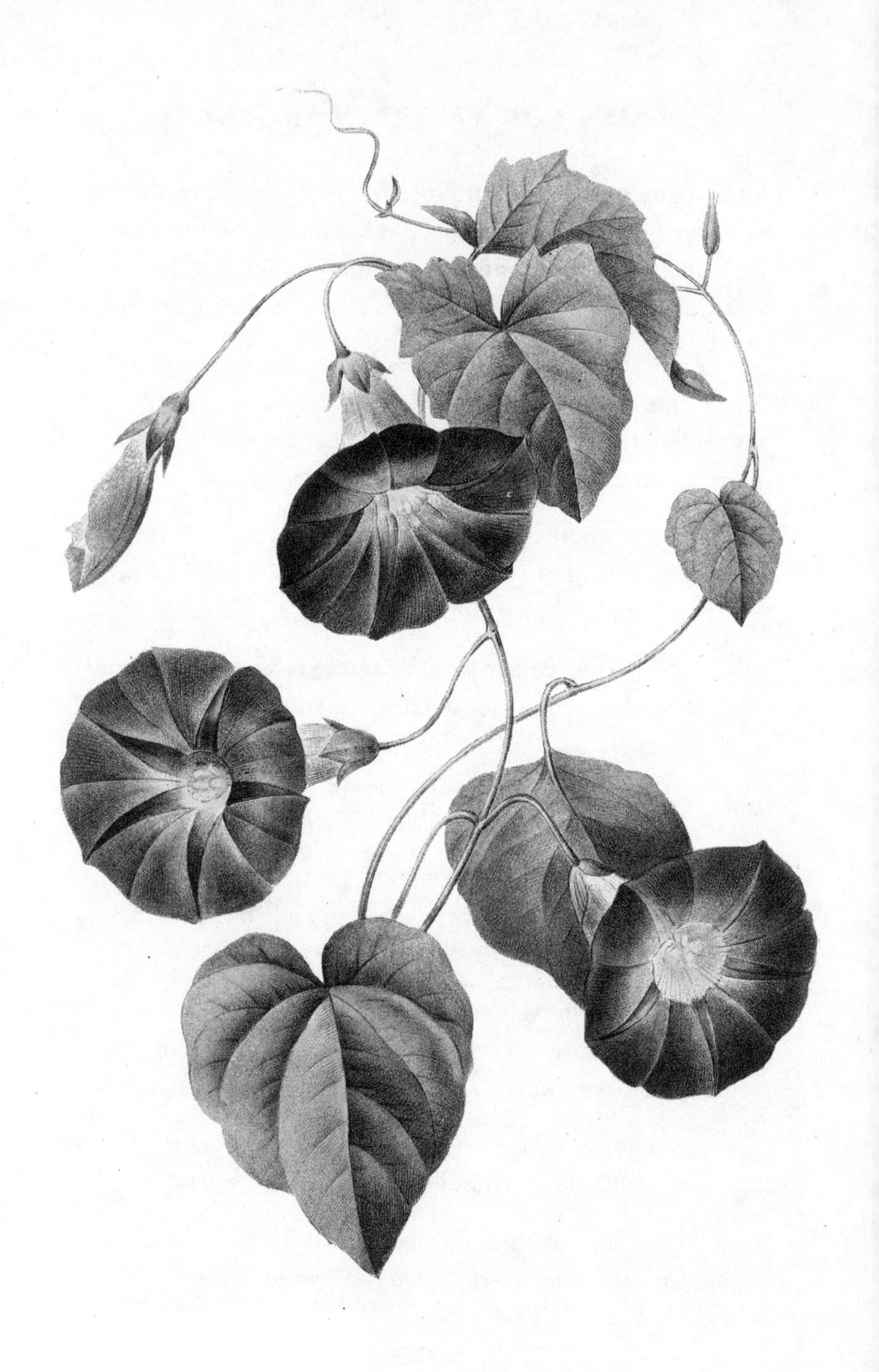

**KARA STANLEY**
with Simon Paradis

# The Pain Project

## A Couple's Story of Confronting Chronic Pain

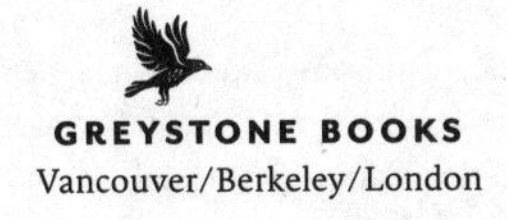

GREYSTONE BOOKS
Vancouver/Berkeley/London

24 25 26 27 28   5 4 3 2 1



Greystone Books Ltd.
greystonebooks.com

Cataloguing data available from Library and Archives Canada
ISBN 978-1-77164-840-0 (pbk.)
ISBN 978-1-77164-841-7 (epub)

Editing by Nancy Flight and Paula Ayer
Proofreading by Alison Strobel
Cover and text design by Jessica Sullivan
Cover illustration (flowers) Pierre-Joseph Redouté, Biodiversity Heritage Library; (nerve) Kohl-Illustration / Alamy Stock Photo

Printed and bound in Canada on FSC® certified paper at Friesens. The FSC® label means that materials used for the product have been responsibly sourced.

Greystone Books thanks the Canada Council for the Arts, the British Columbia Arts Council, the Province of British Columbia through the Book Publishing Tax Credit, and the Government of Canada for supporting our publishing activities.



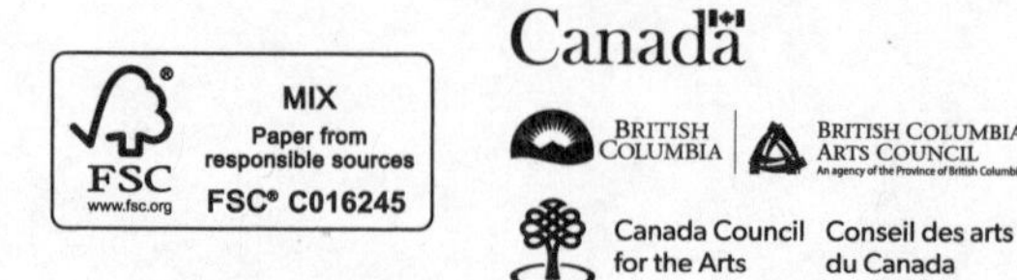


Greystone Books gratefully acknowledges the xʷməθkʷəy̓əm (Musqueam), Sḵwx̱wú7mesh (Squamish), and səlilwətaɬ (Tsleil-Waututh) peoples on whose land our Vancouver head office is located.

# Contents

He has seen but half the universe
who never has been shown the house of Pain.

**RALPH WALDO EMERSON**

*Perfer et obdura, dolor hic tibi proderit olim.*
Be patient and tough;
someday this pain will be useful to you.

**OVID**

# Introduction

IN 2008, MY HUSBAND, SIMON, fell backward off a piece of unsecured scaffold onto stone tile, suffering catastrophic injuries to his brain and spinal cord. In that instant, our world was transfigured. It was an event traumatic enough to shatter any firm notions we held about health, about bad luck and good, about grit and grief and family and the many ways we do—or do not—learn to adapt. Most of all, we had to reconsider everything we thought we knew about pain and the nature of suffering.

The lessons we learned about what we came to refer to as the "indignities of the flesh" were brutal but not uncommon. Most of us will encounter these tough life lessons at some point—preferably in advanced old age—though Simon was only thirty-eight at the time. Before his accident, Simon had been relentlessly, even irritatingly, healthy. In the decade that followed, as his body adjusted to life in a wheelchair, he experienced several life-threatening infections. These were difficult times to negotiate. But even more difficult, more debilitating, was his round-the-clock experience of persistent pain.

Simon's pain imposed significant limits, something we struggled with daily. It was strange, because the severity of Simon's original injuries had already dramatically reshaped our lives. Together we had negotiated a provisional peace with the many permanent consequences of brain and spinal cord injuries. Yet we mightily resisted reconciling ourselves to the seemingly abiding nature of his pain, and we were lost when it came to how best to approach it. Should our focus be on eradicating pain? Or accepting it? Neither option felt entirely right. Focusing on solutions had locked us into a seemingly never-ending, soul-grinding cycle of failed interventions, and we were exhausted. It was increasingly difficult to hold out hope that we'd find an answer. However, accepting that the pain was unsolvable was equally complicated: surely a prerequisite of getting better was a belief that you *could* get better. Would accepting this pain, we asked ourselves, be a gesture of self-fulfilling defeat? If you accept the unacceptable, do you diminish your power to change it?

It was a tough rut to be in: questions without answers; a problem with no solution. Simon's persistent pain was a confounding, paradoxical space, where hope—for the future, for ourselves, for his health—had begun to feel like a potentially dangerous distraction. But the very real prospect of hopelessness? Well, that felt even worse.

A CONSERVATIVE ESTIMATE suggests there are 1.5 billion people—that's one in five people, or 20 percent of the global population—who live in that tough rut of moderate to severe chronic pain, placing an enormous burden on medical systems around the world. Since 1990, low back pain, for example, has consistently been ranked as the number-one health care issue contributing to global disability. Despite this prevalence, the epidemic proportions of pain often go unrecognized. Even though we all know at least one terminally unhappy person who won't stop itemizing the minutiae of their suffering, many people in pain don't like to talk about it. As Simon says, he doesn't "want to lead with his cloud."

Within the medical system, care for people who struggle with chronic pain is fragmented, costly, and contradictory; pain is often either egregiously unrecognized and undertreated or aggressively, even dangerously, overtreated. This situation has resulted in an expensive mess. In Canada, the estimated costs of chronic pain are roughly $60 billion a year. In the U.S., that number is estimated to be somewhere between $560 and $635 billion, an amount that vastly eclipses the annual costs for cancer ($208.9 billion), heart disease and stroke ($363 billion), and diabetes ($327 billion).

Does it help Simon, or me, to know that he isn't alone, that so many others out there are suffering? Nope, not really. Perhaps it even makes it worse. To acknowledge that pain is so universally shared is, well, painful. This, in fact, is persistent pain's superpower: the longer you are in pain, the more sensitive you become. In other words, the more pain you are in the more pain you are in the more pain you are in. It's the mother of vicious cycles.

This book describes the journey that we—Simon and I—undertook in an attempt to disrupt that cycle. Our specific goal was to better understand what the surgeon René Leriche described in 1937 as "living pain"—pain that exists in the everyday world, its scope extending far beyond the confines of hospitals, laboratories, or research articles. Real-world pain is always a humbling experience, and one that is shrouded in profound mystery. When it persists in the absence of a discernable cause, deep suspicion can set in. Physicians, insurers, employers, family members, and friends may doubt the reality of an intangible pain, so much so that the person-in-pain begins to doubt themselves. *What is wrong with me?* they ask. *What did I do to deserve this?* A fine line exists between taking ownership of your individual healing and, even inadvertently, adding to the blame and shame that can pile up as easily as midwinter snowdrifts. Simon and I became preoccupied with this conundrum. Could we discover a place somewhere between hope and hopelessness where we could own, even embrace, the difficult story unfolding in our life?

None of what follows is meant to be prescriptive, and this book does not endorse or discount any given treatment option. What makes pain after spinal cord injury so challenging is that it is resistant to many common interventions. *Intractable* is the word medical professionals use to describe this type of pain, mostly, I think, because that sounds slightly less negative than *incurable.* So, for example, although massage, or steroid injections, or TENS machines (battery-operated devices that deliver small electrical pulses to the body) can be helpful for some people, they had relatively no benefit for Simon. The book we most wanted to write—or read!—was a straightforward guide on how to make the pain stop. But if we have learned nothing else it is this: the scope of the pain experience is complex, and it radically resists a one-size-fits-all approach.

Categorical answers, for the pain sufferer, are hard to come by. This is a difficult truth to face. Still, our marketplaces overflow with promises of surefire cures: a new pill or procedure, a mind-body solution, a guaranteed method to evolve your brain out of pain. It's not that many of these interventions don't have value; they do, usually in combination with one another. But, when it comes to pain, no one solution is surefire: there will always be an exception to the rule. What these ad pitches are really selling is not so much a solution as the illusion of certainty, a promise that if you buy this product, or follow these steps, or join this online program, you can finally stop suffering and rejoin the ranks of the pain-free. The experience of prolonged pain distorts priorities, upends everyday rules of engagement, and imposes its own crooked logic—in this world of extremes, the promise of certainty is fantastically beautiful. It is the mirage wavering on the edge of the desert that leads the parched man to limp on.

Pain sufferers, as Simon and I can attest, will do almost anything to regain a little certainty, even while acknowledging, as we all must, that nothing in life is certain. But the greater the pain endured, the greater the desire for stability in a precarious world. It's easy to make this mirage of certainty our end goal, but in doing so we lose an opportunity to be open and honest about our amazing but vulnerable bodies, subject to the natural world's cycles of renewal and destruction, birth and death. Our bodies, all our bodies, have limits. There is no surefire solution to that.

So Simon and I have abandoned certainty (or perhaps it's more accurate to say that certainty has abandoned us). What we offer instead is a chronicle of the year we chose to accept the challenge posed by pain, a year of few easy answers and many difficult questions. Our goal? To improve our ability to think about how we think about pain. I won't lie; we initially approached our task with some resistance. Certain insights are gained at too high a cost, a fundamental truth that was, in this instance, compounded by the unfair fact that the person who bore the brunt of that cost was not me but Simon. It was tough too in that the close scrutiny of pain is a vast and open-ended endeavor. Not only unique to the person experiencing it, pain is also specific to the time and place and culture in which it is experienced. How we experience pain in our own bodies will influence how we perceive it in others, and vice versa. There are, in fact, so many variables that shape intense pain that, like a tornado or a tsunami, it is a phenomenon that often defies predictive logic.

Ultimately what we learned is this: pain is changeable. Therefore, our understanding of it must also be nimble. As my favorite Toronto Raptor, basketballer Fred VanVleet (aka Steady Freddy), often says: *You can't cheat the process.* And this is the story of *our* process.

### A FEW NOTES ON THE TEXT:

The language Simon and I use to discuss disability and chronic pain has evolved over time, and this is reflected in what follows. The language used in public discourse on these topics is also rapidly changing, and different people may prefer different terms. Our hope is to encourage open discourse and a respect for differences. We believe it is always best to listen first, then honor the ways in which people choose to self-identify.

What follows is an intensely personal tale structured over two years in our married life. However, research for the project spanned a six-year period. Certain timelines have been altered for the sake of maintaining narrative flow. It is, I hope, a forgivable creative liberty, one that has been utilized entirely to enhance the clarity of the content herein.

While not a "How-To" guidebook, *The Pain Project* does aspire to provide you, dear reader, with an expanded toolbox for exploring this difficult topic. To that end, the accompanying endnotes for each chapter provide citations and supplemental information. Additionally, an online Pain Resource Guide (see page 330 for details) offers an expanded discussion on the topic of neuroplastic pain and the importance of movement for the overall health of the nervous system.

Not everything that is faced can be changed;
but nothing can be changed until it is faced.

JAMES BALDWIN

# 1

# An Anniversary

JULY 22, 2018.
*Ten years since Simon's accident.*

I am reading on the porch when Simon cries out from our bedroom. It is a ragged howl, the sound of evisceration, of breath torn from a body.

Another low moan and then rustling sounds as he pulls himself into a seated position. I don't have to see to know exactly what he's doing: bending his torso over his floppy, unfeeling legs in an attempt to stretch out the spasms.

The moan rises in pitch as he transfers from the bed into his wheelchair. He continues to cry out, a kind of frenzied, uncontrolled sob: lawless, utterly disruptive, wholly feral.

Suddenly he calls my name. "Kara!" In an instant, I am on my feet. He never calls for help.

"I'm coming," I say, sprinting into the bedroom. Simon is in the adjoining bathroom, leaning forward in his wheelchair, holding on to the countertop.

"What can I do?" I ask, a familiar thick sense of futility settling in my stomach. I've asked this question so many times before and the answer is always the same.

"Nothing," Simon says. Green eyes gaze at me with a glassy shine, the mobile features of his face—beloved brow, jawline, lips—contorting with another guttural moan. I stand by, useless, as pain carves a new face for him. He exhales and pushes himself into an upright position. "Nothing. There's nothing you can do. You don't have to stay."

"Are you running a fever?"

"No, I don't think so. I just can't catch my breath."

I kneel beside his wheelchair and lean my head into the bony knee of his unfeeling right leg, and he massages the back of my head.

"I'm so sorry, babe," he says.

"Please don't apologize."

"When it's this bad..." he twists my hair in his fingers. "It makes me think that it's nature's way of saying I should never have survived my injuries."

I don't know what to say. There isn't anything to say. I raise my head and draw his hand to my lips, kissing his musician's fingers.

"Song?" he says.

"Sure," I say, feigning enthusiasm. Simply holding the guitar has been setting off spasms lately. I can't imagine him playing a whole song today.

"Okay." He waves me away. "I'll be out in a minute."

SIMON'S PAIN STORY began exactly ten years ago, when he fell off a second-story scaffold and was transported by air ambulance to Vancouver General Hospital. Months later the head neurosurgeon told us that when Simon had arrived in the operating room he was halfway through death's door. I pictured an elegant, wide portal with hardwood accents, tarnished brass fixtures, and stained-glass details. In my mind's eye, Simon leans into the frame, looking back with the particular gaze he saves for me: saucy, inviting. Infrared heat radiating from his smile. Something calls him, but he hovers, undecided. Unwilling, perhaps, to take that final step. Then, with the skilled assistance of a team of surgeons, he steps back into life, and the door, his beautiful death-door, temporarily swings shut.

Pain has been there since the beginning, but—I remind myself again, and again—it hasn't been the whole story. Still, it's hard not to feel otherwise, especially on days like these when the pain, and its effect on our life, looms so large.

After his accident Simon was placed in a medically induced coma. For weeks, his parents and sister joined me in rotating four-hour shifts, spelling each other off at his bedside. Walking the antiseptic hallways under the thrum of fluorescent lights, we lost all sense of night and day. Time slowed, pooling into a deep gully, the dividing line between Before and After. Then and Now.

When Simon was in the ICU I kept a journal that took the form of an open letter, updating him on the dramatic events he was sleeping through. *I left the hospital for forty minutes this afternoon. While I was gone, your heart stopped. Then started again. Now I am afraid to leave the hospital.*

As we moved into the frightening and precarious first year after Simon's accident, I filled a second, then a third journal. Eventually those journals and the accompanying research became a book. It was through the act of writing that I excised the randomness of Simon's accident with the imposition of a beginning, a middle, and (most importantly) an end. At the time, it was important to write a narrative where order was restored, as if by writing it, I could make it so. I wanted to demonstrate that Simon and I could move forward into a full and grateful life despite reckoning with physical infirmities that would have horrified our pre-accident selves.

"Pain," I wrote in the closing pages, "is a powerful teacher of how to live in the present moment." My current feelings regarding that sentence are complicated. It's not that I regret writing it, or that it is untrue. It's more that it is cringeworthy in its naivety and incompleteness.

Pain, I would now add, is boring and obliterative, both. It resists definition. Experienced in the vast inarticulate spaces between one moment of suffering and the next, it resists language. It resists thought. The past and the future fall away. Pain defies everything except its own singularity, trapping you in the present moment.

Approximately three months after Simon's accident, in 2008, he reported a swarming, stinging sensation in his hips, as if he had swallowed a hive of bees that had then nested into the curved bowl of his pelvis. It was significant because the nature of Simon's spinal cord injury—a complete transection of the cord at the L1 and T12 vertebrae—meant he experienced no movement or sensation below his waist. And yet... this.

"There's a buzzing in my bikini line," Simon said, and his physio, Sean, chimed in with a perfectly timed punchline: "Sounds like my college years." We all laughed. At that time, we could still laugh about pain because pain wasn't even close to being our biggest problem. Simon, an inpatient at the GF Strong Rehabilitation Centre, had only recently defied expectations by awaking from his deep comatose state. Doctors had removed the left-side bone plate of his skull to make room for the swelling in his brain, and it was still missing, stored in a freezer at the hospital. I bought a bulky black bike helmet for him to wear as he wheeled down the brightly lit, extra-wide hallways of GF Strong, so there was something more than a thin flap of skin covering his exposed left temporal lobe while we waited for the neurosurgeon to schedule the bone replacement surgery.

There were other issues too: his left arm was unmoving, weaker than a newborn's. He could not transfer in and out of bed on his own but had to be airlifted in a giant sling. He had trouble swallowing and sitting upright in his wheelchair for more than thirty minutes. And the losses stacked up. It wasn't just his legs; he also had no control over his bowels and bladder and no hearing in his right ear. Daily activities were designed to assess the possible deficits in his mental functioning following the brain injury. Pain was an issue, but it was one of many. It was unpleasant, certainly, but also—given the extent of his injuries—reasonable, and we were hopeful that as Simon got stronger and continued to heal, it would fade.

And for the first few months out of rehab, it seemed like that hope was not unfounded. Back at home we booked a weekly physio session, and Simon signed up for a drawing class. Slowly the ability to fret the neck of his guitar with his sleepy left hand returned. Sleeping ten hours every night, he woke every morning stronger than the day before. Spring came, the first in our new accessibly modified home, and we were delighted with the colorful blooms that dotted the yard, the pale violet crocus bravely spearing through the frosty ground. We marked the first anniversary of Simon's accident by planting jasmine in a blue pot on our porch. A few weeks later, after a simple procedure at the podiatrist's, Simon's right big toe developed a form of necrotizing fasciitis, flesh-eating disease, turbo-charged by the antibiotic-resistant superbug MRSA. The absence of pain in Simon's paralyzed limb meant we had no early warning that there was a problem, and by the time we raced into emergency the infection was well established. Six months of intravenous antibiotic drugs followed. The squall of fear and anxiety that had attended his original medical trauma stormed back into our life, and unlike the first time, Simon did not pass through much of it in a comatose state. This time he was awake for it all.

It was Thanksgiving Sunday, three months into our twice-daily intravenous antibiotic routine, when the pain transformed. I was in the kitchen, wrestling with our new, wheelchair-accessible oven. It was the first time I had cooked a turkey in it, and things weren't going well: my organic, free-run, hormone-free—that is to say, ridiculously expensive—bird was charred on top and raw on the bottom. A disaster. Across the room, parked at the kitchen table, Simon cried out, a baffled wail that didn't stop but increased in pitch and intensity.

"What! What is it?" I almost dropped the roasting pan but recovered quickly and managed to shove the bird back in the oven before settling on my knees in front of Simon, who was by turns gasping, moaning, howling. He reached for the kitchen table with his right hand, placed his left on his knee, and looked up at me, eyes damp and bewildered.

"Ow," he said. His comic timing was impeccable, as usual, and he made me smile even as I recognized that he was on the verge of pain-induced tears.

It didn't stop.

Of course, with the sudden spike of pain, we assumed something must be even more radically wrong. Had the MRSA infection spread into his leg bone? Would it need to be amputated? No. Perhaps there was something wrong with the metal rods in his back? Had the infection spread there? A series of urgent appointments and scans followed, none of which provided insight. When, months later, the MRSA infection finally resolved, there was no longer any concrete medical problem for the doctors to fix. Still, the pain raged. Our GP at the time, Dr. James, was a good and kind ally but, like us, had no satisfactory answers. He suggested a higher dose of hydromorphone.

The opioids helped, but only minimally. Simon took them at night, when the pain was at its worst, and his dream life took on a hallucinatory quality. He was convinced that the electrical surges in his hips related to various devices in the house. He would wake me, requesting that I check his computer, or the stereo, believing their electrical circuitry was shorting, and that was what was causing his pain. That was in 2009.

For a time, we were both lost in this new world. The lessons that pain had taught us throughout our lifetime no longer applied. What do you do when acute pain strikes? You seek the source of the problem and take action. You remove yourself from any dangerous stimuli. You assume a posture that will limit further damage and maximize recovery. You promote safety and relief. You give your body adequate time to heal. And when you're ready, you slowly begin to move again.

But Simon's pain was chronic. It was something he lived with constantly, something that altered the microscopic structures of his body, changing him from the inside out. Simon's mysterious agony transported him to a no-man's-land, a kind of living limbo, where there was neither a specific injury to heal nor a place of safety to which he could retreat. After multiple specialist appointments, we were beginning to come to terms with the fact that there was no one authority that could help him.

Simon's paralysis had only underscored how valuable a gift pain truly is. Without pain, he was in constant danger. If he caught his foot in the car door, twisting or even breaking the ankle, he wouldn't immediately feel the hurt of a fractured bone. If, sitting in his wheelchair, he spilled boiling water over his thighs, he wouldn't sense the blistering burns. He didn't experience the mounting discomfort that normally warns us when it's time to shift our position, and that meant the jabbing weight of his own bones could open his skin into horrific, and dangerous, pressure wounds without his noticing. So how, then, could we understand the sizzling, unrelenting pain that surged through these same unfeeling body parts?

I turned to scientific journals, reading everything I could about pain after spinal cord injury. The articles were almost impenetrably dense, pockmarked with graphs and tables, and there was a pervasive lack of consensus regarding certain facts.

There was, however, resounding (and depressing) agreement on a few things. First, pain syndromes associated with stroke and spinal cord injury were examples of a complex chronic pain that rarely if ever resolved, offering a dismally poor prognosis for recovery. Second, spinal cord injury pain was stubbornly resistant to current treatment approaches, which included medications, like gabapentin, and physical treatments, like nerve blocks. Third, chronic pain syndromes affected an extremely high percentage of those who had suffered a spinal cord injury—approximately 61 percent—and the severity of the pain led to several other common complications, such as increased disability, reduced quality of life, depression, and persistent sleep disturbances.

The quandary posed by pain-in-paralyzed-limbs was baffling. The lightning seizures that lit up Simon's body below his level of injury were an implausible, preposterous, cruel taunt of a pain, because, as he said, "It is the only time I have a sense of my legs in space." It was so improbable a type of pain that in the past it was considered impossible. The medical establishment had assumed it to be a kind of sensory illusion: a projection of a neurotic mind unable to cope with the fallout of a catastrophic trauma. Now at least it was recognized as a very real potential outcome of injuries sustained to the spinal cord.

Dr. James retired, and we cycled through a series of young doctors who came to our small coastal town only to leave a year or two later. For the most part, we were on our own. Accustomed to being flexible problem solvers, we struggled to accept that pain, for Simon, was no longer a symptom of an underlying problem but was the disease itself, the consequence of a damaged central nervous system that was wildly misfiring.

"It's like my nervous system is a super-sensitive smoke alarm," Simon said. "Now instead of being triggered by $CO_2$ or billowing smoke or flames, it's going off if I turn the toaster on."

"Yeah," I said. "Or if you have a mild fever."

"Or if I sneeze," Si added. "Or fart. Or move."

"Basically you're setting it off by breathing."

"Fuck." Si shook his head. "Fuck fuck fuck."

Simon decided that ignoring the pain was his best strategy. And why not? Because even though his life, our life, was altered in daily, concrete ways, it seemed that his pain itself was meaningless. There was nothing to do; nothing to fix. *Pain*, we declared to each other, flagrantly appropriating Shakespeare, *is a tale told by an idiot, full of sound and fury, signifying nothing.*

TEN YEARS LATER and we are no closer to truly understanding his pain. It remains a kind of elemental force: an electrical storm, a surging torrent, a continuously crashing wave. References litter the lyrics of Simon's original songs: *There's a pain in the night knows my name*, he writes. *Calls it so sweet and plain. Now I'm all that remains of me.* Music, mercifully, is a buoy that keeps us afloat even on the toughest days. So it's not surprising that on this strange and unsettling anniversary day, Simon emerges from the bedroom still keen to sing a few songs. We start with our version of the jazz standard "Dream a Little Dream of Me," and then I sing "Wagon Wheel." It's an overplayed hootenanny song, but we've come to love it for the simple reason that I can reliably sing it without too many bum notes or instructions from Simon. I have no natural musical gifts, and nothing pains Simon more than making bad music. So I don't suggest working on the harmonies for "Killing the Blues" or the Everly Brothers' "Crying in the Rain." Not today. We don't even make it all the way through "Wagon Wheel": I sing the final recapitulation of the chorus a cappella as Simon, moaning, struggles through a spasm to put the guitar down. But even as his face contorts, he nods at me. "That's good," he says. "Really good. You're right in the center of the note."

Simon is often effusive in his musical praise, but I am almost never the recipient. I'm beaming as I get up to fill the kettle.

"Tea?"

He nods, leaning forward again, pressing his forehead into the edge of the kitchen table, then pushing himself upright, grabbing his right knee, and drawing his thigh to his chest, a violence and urgency to each of these movements. The pain is relentless today.

"I've got to rethink September," Simon says, lowering his leg so that his black sneaker settles in the footrest.

In September, just under two months from now, Si is booked in at Afterlife, the reincarnation of Vancouver's iconic Mushroom Studios. In the spring, he received a Canada Council grant to record an album. For a journeyman musician like Si—so used to making music with relatively little financial support—this is the ultimate: being paid to make an album at a well-equipped studio. He could go on at great length about the near-mystical qualities of the studio's array of mics and pre-amps. I've learned to block out the hours of geeky gear-talk, registering only this crucial fact: Simon is ridiculously excited at the prospect of recording at an established studio with top-notch gear and a dedicated sound engineer.

"I have to cancel. It's too much stress. Too much financial commitment. I can't guarantee my body can handle four days of recording."

"Okay," I say, as the kettle clicks off.

"No tea for me," Si says. "I have to get back into bed."

THE OTHER DAY, Simon was angry with me, and I, in turn, became angry with him. That is unusual for us, especially since his accident. There's not a lot to recommend catastrophic, life-altering injuries, but our shared experience of Simon's trauma continues to teach us, in a very visceral way, the importance of cultivating small gestures of daily kindness. Our anger, when it flares, is rarely directed at each other but rather at the inanities and violence of the world at large. But on that day, it was me Simon was shouting at.

"Stop it!"

I was cutting carrots but, struck by the harshness in his voice, laid my knife down. He had just finished surfing a swell of pain that had caught him as he was opening the fridge door, and now he was glaring at me.

"What?!" I said.

"It's bad enough I have to go through this without you making faces."

"What faces?" Had I been making faces? Maybe I had winced or grimaced? Maybe I had rolled my eyes? If so, it had been involuntary. Simon's pain was such a ubiquitous fixture in our life that I hadn't even registered that particular moment. I had been thinking about what we should make for dinner. "What did I do?"

"Forget it," Simon said, raising a dismissive hand.

"No! No way. Tell me what I did. I have no idea."

"I know." Simon's voice softened. "Forget it, really. I'm sorry."

"Well, talk to me."

A difficult conversation followed. Simon confessed that he felt his pain was having a deep impact on our relationship, and he didn't want it to. I agreed that it was. His world was continuously slowing and narrowing while mine had stayed relatively the same—that is, busy. Busy with work, with household chores, with caregiving duties. Time now moved differently for each of us. Isolated in our own temporal spheres, we both felt distant from each other. Alone.

Neither of us wanted Simon's pain to be the driving force in our life, but it was. It had been for years. Simple touching, my hand or my head resting on his shoulder, was often too much for him to bear. Every few hours throughout the night, pain interrupted his sleep, and consequently mine. The resulting fatigue severely limited his ability to work and, to a lesser degree, mine as well. Having dinner with friends on the weekend was generally more of a commitment than we could make. I confessed to hating how powerless his pain made me feel. We both confessed to feeling, underneath our soothing daily rituals and shared acts of kindness, angry, sad, and lonely. And despairing, because there was no end in sight.

"I don't know what I did, just now, making a face, or whatever. And you know the last thing I want to do is make it worse for you. But as much as you might feel alone, I am living this right beside you. And when you howl? It affects my body too. I need room to wince or sigh."

"I know. I'm sorry. This isn't the life I wanted for you." Si's usually animated facial expressions were flat. He was so exhausted. Years-of-sleepless-nights exhausted. It took such strength for him to get up every morning, but that strength—I could see in his pale face—was running out.

"It's not what I want for you either," I said, deeply apprehensive of what one of us might say next. As good as it was to say these words out loud, it felt as though we were on the precipice of freeing a devastating truth into our lives. I leaned over and kissed his forehead. "You know, I'm not sure talking about this helps."

"Right?" Simon said. "There's something to be said for keeping it all bottled up."

Neither of us believed that, but at the same time, it felt true. Some things once said can't be ignored.

"Dinner?" he asked. "Then do you want to watch a movie?"

NOW, A FEW DAYS LATER, the silence of those unsaid words has only grown louder. As Si naps through the balmy afternoon, I once again escape to the warm cedar planks of our porch. Chico, our dog, settles down beside me, afternoon light glinting copper in his chestnut coat. I call our son, Eli, who at twenty-five is working hard to build his own life in Vancouver. Catching him during a busy workday, I strive to keep the call short, upbeat, realizing the moment I hear his voice how unfair it would be to tell him the truth: that I miss him and wish he were here to help us move through this difficult day. Preoccupied with a hectic afternoon schedule, he is blissfully unaware that this is the anniversary of Simon's accident, and for this I'm thankful. It would be an unkindness to remind him. "I love you," I say instead, signing off.

Up above the sky is an untroubled blue. The cooling breeze carries the signature bouquet of a Pacific Northwest summer: salt-smudged ocean and sun-toasted cedar. But even this glorious weather can't fend off a descending sense of dread, or the sudden certainty that it is not us but the pain that has triumphed. Chico nudges his nose against my shoulder, eyebrows wrinkling into a lazy question.

"It's okay, buddy," I say. "Simon will be fine. We'll be fine."

Satisfied, he plops back down, stretching over onto his back, legs indiscreetly splayed: time for a belly rub.

I wish I could be so easily convinced. But the heartbreaking reality I have been wrestling with all day is that, impossible as it seems, somehow the pain has become worse over, what, the past year? Maybe two? Simon simply has no more push left. And unchecked, this pain appears to be boundless. Like Nigel Tufnel's amp in *Spinal Tap,* it keeps turning up to eleven. It's become tough to talk about the situation with friends and family; the words I say—*he's going through a rough patch, his pain is really bad right now*—have become repetitious, and somehow shameful.

Simon re-emerges from the bedroom as I am serving dinner: salmon, asparagus, and new potatoes. Before we eat, we make a toast.

"To surviving," Simon says.

"'Anniversary' is such a strange word under the circumstances," I say. "Too celebratory. Maybe 'commemoration' is better?"

Simon nods. "It's been quite the decade."

"Yeah. Listen, Beau—" I say.

"Uh-oh," he interrupts. "You always call me Beau when you're pitching an idea you know I'll hate."

"Not true! It's a term of endearment." My indignation rings disingenuous, and he raises his eyebrows, waiting for me to continue. "Okay, yes, fine. You're right. I am about to make an unpleasant pitch. But . . . we have to do something."

"Ahhh . . . okay. About what?"

"About the pain. I want my husband back."

"Hey!" He looks at me directly, hurt. "That's not fair. I'm right here."

"I know. I'm sorry. But it's as if the pain is stealing all your agency. And I miss *you*. Do you know what I mean? Is that fair to say?"

"Yeah." Simon sighs. "I'm always exhausted. I miss me too."

"We can't keep doing the same things and expect anything will get better. It doesn't work and it's crazy-making."

"Maybe it won't get better," Simon says. "What then?"

"What if I take time off work and we tackle it head-on?" I ask, for the moment ignoring his challenge. "Review the research. Revisit our past pain-intervention strategies. Rethink our diet. Recommit to daily exercise. I'll write about it. You write about it. It'll be our own personal experiment. Together, a kind of joint quest."

"Hhmmmmpfh." Simon extends the unhappy syllable long enough to let me know that he knows I'm insisting on only one answer to this invitation. After twenty-plus years of marriage, I read the subtext of his skeptical face clearly: *Your big plan will mean a boatload of work for me and will likely include a lot of flaky bullshit like guided meditations and increasing our daily dose of fermented foods, and I—didn't you just hear me?—am already fucking exhausted.*

"Please," I say.

"Okay," he says.

# 2

# Introducing Rupert

JULY 23, DAY I.

What, exactly, is pain? This is a question we have been asking for ten years. And it's where we start today, on the first day of our TACKLING PAIN project.

"Can we always say it like this," I ask Simon. "In all caps, or like a UFC announcer?" I lower my voice an octave. "Defending champion Simon Paradis faces down his challenger, PAAAAAIN."

My attempts at being lighthearted are not appreciated. Simon shoots me a brief glare before parking his wheelchair at the kitchen table. Unwrapping the plastic on the black Moleskine journal I bought him, he sighs theatrically: "This feels like the first day of school."

"Right?!" I say. I loved the first day of school.

"You're nuts, Stanley." He picks up a pen and opens the journal to that first, inviting, blank page. "Okay. What next?"

"Well," I say, opening my matching journal. "We should probably start at the beginning."

Simon nods, then scribbles down a quick sentence.

*What is pain?*

IT DOESN'T MATTER how many times you ask, it's always a difficult question to answer. The word *pain* itself is both too big and too small: too broad at its borders; too insufficient in its intimate details. Pain is an amorphous shapeshifter, the wily companion to cancer treatments, collapsed lungs, and stubbed toes; bruised elbows and bruised egos. Headaches and heartaches. The vastly different experiences of a sprained ankle, giving birth, and sensing the agonized presence of a phantom limb all rely upon this single word—*pain*—to convey a kaleidoscope of meaning. Despite being ubiquitous in everyday life, pain is slippery. Both a universal aspect of the human condition and an experience that is uniquely individual, pain, Simon and I have discovered, has a perverse tendency to flout tidy borders.

Understanding pain is even more difficult than defining it, and not just for us. "The relief of pain is obviously one of the main functions of physicians," psychiatrist Frank Ervin said in 1959. "Ironically, it's one of the things we do least well—partly because we don't understand it." Flash forward sixty years to the findings of a review of pain education in ten Canadian universities in the faculties of medicine, nursing, dentistry, pharmacology, physical therapy, occupational therapy, and veterinary medicine: while the veterinary students were two to five times more likely to receive pain education than the health science students, a whopping 68 percent of all programs had no designated hours devoted to the topic.

Internationally the picture is no better. In the U.K. and U.S., 96 percent of medical schools have no compulsory teaching curriculum dedicated to pain medicine. The median number of hours dedicated to pain content for the average medical student is eleven in the U.S., twelve in European countries, and thirteen in the U.K. Canada, Australia, and New Zealand are on the high end, offering a median of twenty hours, or about 0.4 percent of the total teaching hours required to earn a medical degree. Primary care physicians around the world express a lack of preparedness to provide optimal care for patients with pain, citing their limited training and lack of confidence in their ability to provide effective treatment. "Acute, chronic and cancer pain remain ineffectively managed," concluded a systematic review of pain medicine content in international medical school curricula, "partly as a result of a lack of expertise of medical practitioners."

Pain—especially the human kind—is still not understood all that well; wherever they are in the world, most people entering the health care system will be treated by a physician who does not have specialized training in pain medicine.

The International Association for the Study of Pain defines pain as "an unpleasant sensory and emotional experience associated with, or resembling that associated with, actual or potential tissue damage." Nietzsche, who suffered injuries during a horseback-riding accident that only intensified a lifelong propensity for migraines, famously named his pain "dog," a vivid linguistic attempt to domesticate the unruly forces of suffering in his life. Patrick Wall, one of the great innovators of modern pain science, suggested we view pain as a "need state" that, like hunger or thirst, requires a specific action (a pill, or a procedure, or a kiss on the boo-boo by a parent—any action, really, that returns the sufferer to a state of perceived safety) to assuage it. One of my favorite chapters in Marni Jackson's excellent book *Pain: The Fifth Vital Sign* characterizes pain as an odious bore, an unwelcome dinner guest who drives a Ford Taurus and picks his teeth with a shish kebab skewer, all the while directing a braying monologue at the author.

"No, what is true (Pain argues) is that you're alone in this body, feeling its borders and contours as a constant, mild, and grievous ache," Jackson writes. "Pain electrifies the fence between you and the rest of the world."

This passage echoed in my mind long after I finished the book because it felt both right and wrong in relation to Simon and me. The right: *an electrified fence*. Simon's pain is like a hideous fence, festooned with barbed wire, the current so powerful you can sense its pulsing heat if you hold the palm of your hand six inches from its surface. It separates us. The wrong: *a constant, mild, and grievous ache*. I'm familiar with that type of pain. We all are. It's the pain of pulled muscles after an intense workout, or of a work week (or month, or year) that has demanded more and more and then still more of you. Perhaps it's the pain of flu just about to break, or pain that is a preview of the stiffening joints of old age. It's the kind of pain for which I feel a sense of gratitude, because it's a sensation that can be moved through.

But Simon is handcuffed to that hideous fence, and even the hint of a supportive gesture, say, my hand brushing his shoulder, only amps up the voltage. He has invisible jumper cables attached to his hips, jolting him, sometimes from a deep sleep, with their electric current. Our son, Eli, at seventeen, had said that living with Simon's pain was like living with a wolf caught in a leg trap. It is an uncompromising state of being.

I relay Jackson's description of her unwanted dinner guest to Simon, and he too is delighted. The Ford Taurus is the perfect touch. And Simon can relate: for years, he has personified his pain as an angry child. "What's his name?" I ask now.

"Rupert."

"He's British?"

"Possibly. Snotty, definitely. A real asshole."

"Why is he angry?"

"Oh man," Simon says. "Why *isn't* he angry?"

MARNI JACKSON'S BOOK, so expansive in both its compassion and intelligence, underscored the difficult lesson that Simon and I have spent the last decade learning and relearning: pain is complicated. Really, really complicated. It's complicated in the way that seemingly simple things may be, like, say, how does a bike work? Or, why are yawns contagious? It's also complicated in a deeply mysterious way, as challenging as understanding the concept of quantum entanglement, or the impenetrable nature of dark matter. But, mostly, pain is complicated in the way that the arguably most complicated thing in the known universe—the human brain—is, and this is because pain is always a creation of the brain.

Initially, Simon was affronted when I brought this basic maxim of current pain research to his attention, violently rejecting the notion that his pain was, in some way, imaginary. But saying that pain is a creation of the brain is not the same thing as saying that it is imaginary.

What it means is that pain is your nervous system's way of alerting you that something is wrong. It means that different parts of your body are constantly sending alerts to your brain for interpretation, and if your brain decides there is a credible threat of harm, it will create pain. *Real* pain. This is true even if your brain is being bombarded with bad information, as it is for Simon. Overloaded with these danger signals, the brain—that industrious and protective overseer—will amp up a pain response, even in the absence of actual threat.

When Simon and I first discussed this years ago, he had said, "So. My legs don't work; my bowels and bladder don't work; and now... my brain is hijacking me? And how does knowing this help? It's the ultimate betrayal."

It was a perspective I'd never considered, and I realized (not, sadly, for the first or last time) how little I truly understood of what Simon faced each day.

We have continued to talk about this axiomatic truth about pain over the years, volleying ideas back and forth as our understanding grew. Pain literature repeatedly underscores this central point: pain does not become pain until it reaches the conscious, thinking part of your brain. General anesthetic, for example, works because it separates the evolutionarily ancient, automatic, survival part of the brain from the more recently developed thinking, perceiving, feeling parts. Under anesthesia, your survival brain remains active (so you don't die), but danger signals arriving from the outer parts of the body are blocked from reaching your chemically muted conscious brain. This is what allows a surgeon to slice deep into skin and muscle, scoop out an appendix, and stitch you back up, all without a whimper or a moan.

"Okay," Simon said when I offered up this example. "Still, I don't like it. Saying pain is all in your brain, it's... unkind."

"It's not kind, or unkind," I said. "It's science. It's a fact."

"When your mom died and you were sad, did I comfort you by saying, 'This grief you're feeling—it's all in your brain'? No. That might be a fact too, but it would also be a stupid and cruel thing to say to a grieving person."

"Okay. But if that grief became entrenched, lasting for years, or decades, wouldn't it be appropriate to have some kind of intervention? To recognize that your brain has become stuck in a certain way of seeing and being in the world?"

Simon grunted in reply.

"Am I being stupid and cruel?" I asked.

"No. Of course not," he said. "But I'm not sure you totally get how the statement *pain is in the brain* makes me feel. You think it's interesting, hopeful even. Me, I'm suddenly an abandoned kid tossed out into the street. I can't trust my body; I can't trust my brain. I'm orphaned. Homeless."

"That's a horrible way to feel," I said.

"You're telling me, sister."

IT WAS EARLY ON, when Simon was in rehab after his accident, that we both became familiar with the three broad medical classifications of bodily pain: nociceptive, neuropathic, and neuroplastic.

The first, **nociceptive**, is the most common and is what most of us would refer to as acute pain. This pain is present when the tissues of the body have been damaged, or when damage is about to occur. Part of the intricate network of peripheral nerves, nociceptors are specialized receptors that respond to all potentially damaging stimuli. If we sit still for too long, nociceptors cue us to get up and move around. If a finger strays too near an open flame, or gets pinched in a car door, nociceptors warn us to take immediate action (pull the hand back, open the door) to limit damage.

For example, if you were to twist your ankle, the membranes of the nociceptors would stretch and bend unpleasantly, initiating an immediate electrochemical message to the brain about a new potential threat to the body. And the brain, operating at a speed much faster than conscious thought, would also send a steady stream of information about appropriate ways to respond. If you're crossing the street when the ankle twist occurs, your brain might decide that you need to get safely out of traffic, sit down, and rest your foot while further assessing the damage. However, if instead you're frantically outmaneuvering a grizzly bear, your brain will have an entirely different message, more along the lines of *Help! Fuck! There's a bear chasing me!* The brain will not prioritize an achy ankle until the other, greater, danger has passed.

This lightning-fast conversation between the peripheral nerves and the brain has several junctures in the spinal cord—most commonly imagined as "gates"—that, depending on the situation, modulate the nociceptors' warning. In the first scenario where you twist your ankle, your brain might assess the incoming nociceptive message as highly important: the "gates" in the spinal cord will open, increasing the nociceptive signal and amplifying your discomfort. The ankle might feel hot or swollen almost immediately, not to mention the searing pain radiating up your leg with every step you take. But in the second scenario, when the nociceptors shout their warning—*Attention! Strained ankle*—the brain will respond to this lesser threat (Strained ankle? Pish. There's a BEAR!) with an inhibitory signal, closing the gates.

In this situation, paying attention to your ankle diminishes your chances of survival, so the brain, in all its wisdom, temporarily shuts that warning signal down.

Congenital insensitivity to pain with anhidrosis, or CIPA, is an extremely rare genetic condition in which a person is born without the capacity to feel pain. While a pain-free life might sound fabulous, it generally isn't. People with this condition are constantly at risk of life-threatening injuries. They rarely escape childhood without a horrible litany of wounds—burns, lacerations, tips of tongues bitten off while chewing food, burst appendixes, and broken bones—and their life expectancy is far lower than average. But aside from the folks in this exclusive group, we are all familiar with nociceptive pain.

Less common is **neuropathic** pain, or pain that results when injured nerves send misleading or excessive signals to the rest of the nervous system. This type of damage may occur for many reasons, including physical trauma (as in Simon's case), stroke, a genetic condition or degenerative disease, or infection such as shingles. It can cause profound changes in the way pain is perceived: things that hurt before now hurt more (a state known as hyperalgesia), and things that didn't hurt before now do (a state known as allodynia). Normal sensations—even a light touch or the weight of a flannel sheet—can become excruciatingly painful.

The third type of pain, **neuroplastic** (or **nociplastic**), results when the nervous system responds to a protracted state of pain by making adaptations in how it processes this sensation. Overloaded with information and unable to regulate this barrage effectively, the nervous system becomes increasingly sensitized. When pain becomes chronic, it generally has a neuroplastic component. This makes it incredibly difficult to address, because while this pain is always felt in a specific body part (the low back, or a shoulder, or the neck), it is not just the low back or shoulder or neck that requires healing but also the nervous system itself.*

Adding to the complexity is the fact that the boundaries of these three types of pain are not rigid; they tend to blur and tangle in a complicated way. Simon, for example, experienced nociceptive pain in the aftermath of the fall that fractured his skull bones and vertebrae. Neuropathic pain, too. The central nervous system is composed of the brain, the brain stem, and the spinal cord, and Simon sustained significant damage in all three of these areas. When his spinal cord was severed, changes occurred within the entire nervous system, not just at the original site of injury, and these changes caused the metaphorical gates—those junctures in the spinal cord that modulate the sensation of pain—to be blown wide open. Inhibitory signals (that reduce pain) were decreased while excitatory signals (that amplify pain) proliferated. And when this pain-storm didn't stop, his neuroplastic nervous system began to adapt, becoming more reactive to any perceived threat.

Simon has a favorite phrase to describe disputes that have reached a state of irreconcilable differences. "Two icebergs," he says. "No ship." And that's how I sometimes think of his pain: as a conversation between his central and peripheral nervous system that has become—like his spinal cord—catastrophically disconnected. Before his accident, both

* Visit the online Pain Resource Guide (see page 330) for an expanded discussion on the potential indicators that pain is neuroplastic in nature and possible ways to address it.

Simon and I had always understood pain as a symptom of some other, underlying issue. But now pain itself was the issue. Within this new equation, it helped to conceive of the complicated cocktail of nociceptive, neuropathic, and neuroplastic pain as a disease. We started adding key qualifiers to label his pain: *persistent*, *centralized*, *chronic*. Changing our language didn't diminish the intensity of his experience, but it did lessen our panic.

And lessening our panic helped, a bit. But as time wore on we also began to understand that further complicating these three categories of pain was the reality that when extreme pain persists long enough it transforms into something altogether new: suffering. Pain was a problem of the body. But suffering? That was a malady of the soul.

PAIN, WE ALSO LEARNED, always has a context. The intensity, duration, and distress of pain are influenced by a vast array of factors, some we may be aware of but many we are not. Your physical and mental health at the time of injury is important, as are your attitudes, memories, and beliefs about injury and pain. It matters if you have a supportive network surrounding you while you heal, or if the injury and prospective pain affects your financial stability. The exact same injury can affect two people with different health profiles, histories, or economic situations in dramatically different ways.

Various studies—some that can only be described as deviously clever, for surely the pain researchers were having a little fun at their subjects' expense—demonstrate the many, often oddball, factors that can influence the perception of pain. Is the person administering the test wearing a white coat and carrying a clipboard or otherwise presenting as a figure of medical authority? Or is it just some regular schmo? Is the test subject given a detailed explanation of what to expect in the experiment, or no explanation at all? Is the pain-generating stimulus accompanied by bad smells? Or sounds of extreme distress?

These factors along with others, such as the test subject's satisfaction with their work or their spousal relationship or a previous history of painful experiences, will affect the subject's assessment of pain. According to different studies, colored pills work better for pain relief than plain white ones, a capsule filled with multicolored beads works better yet, and an injection works best of all. Amazingly, this hierarchy of effectiveness remains the same whether the medication is a traditional pharmaceutical pain reliever or a placebo.

One sneaky research study applied a painfully cold stimulus to participants' forearms. Overwhelmingly the participants self-reported a higher pain level when the stimulus was accompanied by a red light as opposed to a blue light, although the intensity of the stimulus remained the same. The researchers theorized that the red light was associated with a state of emergency or danger, a cognitive association strong enough to influence the participants' perception of the intensity of the sensation.

Over the past few centuries, the theater of war has provided real-world research into this mercurial nature of pain. Military medics have repeatedly observed that men wounded in battle do not react to serious injuries in a predictable manner, but it wasn't until Lieutenant Colonel Henry Beecher, an army anesthesiologist during World War II, documented the reactions of 215 severely wounded soldiers that a plausible explanation for this was put forward. Even though the soldiers' injuries were calamitous—gunshot wounds, amputations, compound fractures—they demonstrated incredible stoicism. Of the wounded, only 33 percent required painkillers. In contrast, 80 percent of a group of civilians with similarly severe injuries requested narcotics.

Beecher determined that the soldiers were not in a state of shock that made them unable to experience pain. They complained when a nurse awkwardly inserted a needle, so clearly their fortitude had limits. Nor could Beecher find any dependable relationship between the extent of the wounds and the intensity of pain experienced. He concluded that the only significant difference between the soldiers and the civilian group was what the pain meant. For civilians, catastrophic injury could mean a whole host of crappy outcomes: loss of work, financial instability, increased vulnerability, the prospect of a lifelong disability. For soldiers, an injury meant permanent retreat from the battlefield. The hospital was a place of relative safety. A serious injury also meant they would be returning home. Their active duty was over. Beecher hypothesized that the soldiers' strong emotions—joy, euphoria, relief—acted as an anodyne to the troubles of the flesh.

Physical pain is often accompanied by some correlating issue in the tissues of the body. Over time, the resilience of certain tissues may have diminished, due to injury, inflammation, or delayed healing. This has led to the belief that there is a straightforward relationship between tissue damage and pain: the greater the tissue damage, the greater the pain. Plenty of examples appear to demonstrate that truth. A stab wound, for example, will likely hurt more throughout its healing process than, say, a paper cut. But in the annals of pain history, an abundance of real-life, anecdotal, and researched evidence clearly demonstrates the correlation is not at all straightforward. Even the above example is tricky. As anyone who has sliced their finger chopping vegetables or stepped on sharp glass knows, a deep, clean wound usually announces itself with a bloom of blood, not a stab of pain, whereas a paper cut immediately results in an insistent, aggravating sting.

Pain and tissue damage are related, but they are not the same thing.

Along with the reports of medical men like Colonel Beecher that noted the strange lack of correlation between severity of injury and perceived pain in soldiers, there are countless other examples of people who suffer significant tissue damage but experience little or no pain. These stories often center on acts of great athletic endurance (the hockey player who scored the winning Stanley Cup goal with a fractured hand), exceptional heroism (the mother who pulled her child from a burning vehicle despite her own second-degree burns), or extreme self-preservation (the man who swam fifty yards to escape a great white shark, then discovered the knock he felt to his midriff was, in fact, a gaping abdominal wound).

But no story more dramatically illustrates the complicated relationship between tissue damage and perceived pain than the one described in a now oft-cited 1995 column in the *British Medical Journal*. A twenty-nine-year-old British construction worker—let's call him Oliver—arrived at the emergency department after jumping onto a six-inch nail. Included in the article is a grainy black-and-white photo of a well-worn work boot pierced with a nefariously long nail that entered through the rubber sole and exited through the leather top.

When Oliver arrived at the hospital, he was apparently in agony. Tiny jostles, or attempts to touch the nail, caused him even greater distress, and so doctors administered a powerful cocktail of fentanyl and midazolam. Oliver relaxed enough that they could extract the nail and remove the boot. Amazingly, the foot was uninjured, the nail having slid between the young man's sweaty toes.

Pain experts like to relate this story to make the point that even in the absence of tissue damage, the brain can create significant pain. It's a difficult, counterintuitive thought. But after we're done rolling our eyes at poor hysterical Oliver and making our snap judgments (he must have been a whiner from the get-go, mustn't he?), we should remind ourselves of the times when the anxious narrator in our own mind has told such a convincing story of fear and threat that our discomfort vastly eclipsed what was appropriate to the situation. How many of us, at one time or another, have feared that a severe headache indicated a brain tumor or that a stomachache was a sure sign of bowel cancer? No matter where you fall on the personality spectrum—tending toward anxiety and neurosis, like me, or a confident extrovert, like Simon—I'm certain you have at least one story like that of your own. I sympathize with poor Oliver; when the fentanyl buzz wore off and he learned of his unharmed foot, he must have been mortified.

The *BMJ* story leaves many questions unanswered. Had Oliver, for example, recently witnessed a construction site accident that caused devastating injuries to a coworker? Or was he a new father, with a wife and baby at home who were depending on him and his work wages? Possibly he was a stoic fellow, prone to ignoring the discomfort from an undiagnosed stomach ulcer that had been acting up all day. Speculative questions only, because we will never know the circumstances of that particular day, for that particular British builder. Oliver's extreme reaction will remain a mystery because we have no context in which to situate the sudden pain he felt when he saw the nail piercing the leather of his boot. But pain always has a context. Pain in the present relates intimately to both the lessons of our past and our expectations of the future. It is always highly conditional, varying not just from person to person but from situation to situation.

Here's the million-dollar question, though: Was the pain Oliver felt *real*?

According to current theories of pain perception, the answer is yes. When Oliver's brain perceived a significant threat to his body, it activated—at a speed much faster than conscious thought—an integrated global defense designed to reduce further harm. Along with the agonizing sensation in his foot, most likely Oliver's heart pounded, his blood pressure soared, and his breath came in short, ragged gasps. Adrenaline coursed; white blood cells rallied, and his body temperature might have begun to rise, anticipating infection invading his bloodstream. For Oliver, perceived threat was enough to shift all these biological systems into high gear. The reliable indicator of pain in this situation was not tissue damage but the brain's perception of the body's state of jeopardy.

The idea that the brain has its own convictions, priorities, and agenda for the body was one I became familiar with early in Simon's recovery while reading the work of neuroscientist V. S. Ramachandran. One of his many insights resulted in the mirror-box experiment, an elegant, low-cost attempt to address the "phantom limb" sensations of an amputated arm. Some people experience devastating pain in their missing limb, but for others the ghostly sensations are even more puzzling: agonizing itches or burning, clenched hands, arms frozen in troubling positions. Like pain sensed in paralyzed limbs, phantom limb sensations present a perplexing conundrum. How do you address issues in a limb that is no longer physically present? Ramachandran's solution was to build a simple structure with two holes in the front and a vertical mirror running through the middle, allowing a volunteer to "place" their phantom limb behind the mirror and the unharmed arm in front. In this way, the reflected image of the working arm created an impression that both arms were restored and functional. Through this visual trompe l'oeil, people could address some of the strange manifestations of their phantom limbs: arms could gesture and wave, hands could open and close, itches were scratched. The mirror illusion restored a visual sense of physical wholeness, and often pain was reduced.

The brain's perceptions are powerful but also imperfect, vulnerable to being tricked or manipulated. Because Simon's pain—the electrical zaps and blooms and spasms—all happen below his injury, in an area where he has neither sensation nor movement, the comparison to phantom limb pain is apt. Simon's pain, at least partly, is a kind of ghost in the machine, a terrible and punishing sensory hallucination.

BACK AT THE KITCHEN TABLE, both our journals remain blank save for that taunting question: *What is pain?*

"I know you hate the 'pain is a product of the brain' phrase. And the last thing I want is to make you feel abandoned, or homeless, but can we agree," I ask Simon now, "that the brain, in response to various incoming messages from the body, is responsible for creating the sensation of pain? That this is our most reasonable point of departure?"

"I don't know. To me, it still sounds like a complicated way of saying the pain is all in my mind."

"Well," I say. "It kind of is."

"Fuck off," he says, but not in a mean way.

"Look, we both know your pain is very real. Of course it's not all in your mind."

"But is there really a difference?" Simon asks. "Between saying pain is made by the brain or that it's all in your mind?"

"Well, yeah. They might be used interchangeably, but 'brain' and 'mind' are not the same thing."

A brief digression follows as we discuss the difference between *brain*, an organ weighing approximately three pounds housed within the skull, and *mind*, a vague term that encompasses key aspects of the brain's cognitive functions: perceiving, remembering, evaluating, predicting, deciding. Humanity is still undecided on the most fundamental of chicken-or-egg questions: Does the brain create the mind? Or does the mind create the brain? Are our thoughts, actions, and health profiles entirely a by-product of our unique physiological makeup, our personalities bubbling up out of our specific electrochemical stew? The world of science tends to prefer this lens, viewing any mind-talk as wildly imprecise. Flaky, even. But most of us intuitively resist such a deterministic outlook, preferring a perspective where, through the functions of the mind—thinking, feeling, choosing—we have agency to shape not only our personal destinies but our bodies as well.

"This is the kind of conversational side street that would have felt profound when you were eighteen, sitting at the kitchen table sipping whiskey at the end of a long party night," Si says. "But bottom line, no one really knows who's driving the bus—brain? Or mind? And common sense says it's never either-or but a mix of both."

"Agreed. For us, I think the important thing to remember is that *mind* refers solely to conscious, cognitive functions. But the brain is always working at both the conscious and unconscious level. Cognitive stuff but also immune stuff, hormone stuff. Heart rate. Blood pressure. Respiration," I say. "Maybe your issue with the statement 'pain is a product of the brain' is a problem of language. Would it help if we said 'pain is made by your nervous system'? Does that feel better?"

"Yeah." Simon shrugs. "It does. More accurate."

"Maybe *made* is the wrong word too."

"What about *translated* or *interpreted*?" Simon suggests. "Pain is translated by your nervous system."

"Right!" I say. "The nervous system interprets information from inside and outside the body, translating it, or not, into the experience of pain. Does that work for you?"

"Yeah." Simon nods. "I can live with that."

We decide that the first action in our TACKLING PAIN project is to momentarily forget all the clinical definitions and write, in our brand-new journals, what pain means to us right now. At the end of ten minutes we exchange notebooks, and Simon reads my words out loud:

*Our current experience of pain is one in which all order is lost. Forward progress has been replaced by an unending series of jabbing, bewildering attacks upon Simon's body. It is the ultimate chaos narrative. Simon and I have been wading in the murky waters of this chaos story the past few years. I hate it. Every day pain pushes Simon from the shore of our daily life, out to open sea. There is nothing I can do but wave my arms and call for help. Simon, who is always more attentive to my welfare than his own, tries to ease my distress by cracking one-liners, or belting out a version of Bowie's "Moonage Daydream." Still, he moves further and further away, his voice growing fainter.*

Simon looks up from the page. "Whoa, Stan. That's heavy." He smiles, a dreamboat of a smile, unchanged from the first time I basked in its warmth, thirty-three years ago, when we met in grade ten history class. "Maybe a little dramatic?"

"I don't know. To me, it feels like I've understated the drama of when you're screaming in pain."

"Fair enough. I'm sorry."

"Don't apologize." I pick up his notebook and read:

*Pain, for me, is like an impetuous, domineering, insistent weather front. And I'm the farmer endlessly trying to make his land fertile again, but I'm hijacked at every stage. Hurricanes come, mess up the tilling. Late frosts come, mess up the planting. Monsoons come, mess up the harvest. And at any moment locusts might descend or a firestorm might be ignited, messing up everything. Over time the soil gets so depleted nothing will ever grow there again.*

Errant tears flood my gaze, the words on the page blurring. "Oh, Beau," I say, looking up. "I'm so sorry."

"Now, don't you apologize," he says, handing me a Kleenex. "Okay. What next?"

"Well—"

"Wait a sec." He holds up a hand, fending off any of my suggestions. "I have a gig in two weeks. Pain stuff will have to wait."

"Maybe you could do a little journaling?"

"Hmmm. We'll see. And let me guess, you'll start with some... reading?"

"Yeah," I say and blithely begin listing off the books, journals, and pain organizations I'm planning to investigate. The list is long and I am enthusiastic, and so it takes me a minute to realize that Simon is tapping his pen against his lips, shaking his head, and laughing. "Sorry," I say, interrupting myself mid-sentence. "I guess it's unseemly to be so enthused about embarking on Pain School."

"*Kara Stanley's School of Pain*. Not as fun as a School of Rock, and definitely open to some sketchy interpretations," Simon says, still laughing. "But it's perfect. I love it."

# 3

# An Action Plan

OCTOBER 5, DAY 75.

Long days of lazy sunlight draw out a warm September, but by October autumn arrives with a briny, windswept fury. Yellow leaves plaster the forest floors; atmospheric rivers of rain roll in off the Pacific; and power lines are routinely knocked down. Once again we're dining by candlelight. A gust of wind buffets the window pane and the flame flickers in response, shadows cavorting across the ceiling.

The power has been out all day and the house is cold. I'm wearing my wool hat and two pairs of socks, and we've wrapped Simon's icy legs in a sheepskin blanket. It's the third time in two weeks that we're eating canned lentil soup (an easy meal to prepare in the dark), and once again the plan is to crawl into bed on the shy side of eight o'clock. This is a routine that quickly grows tiresome, but I also love it. The silence in the absence of computers, phones, or TV leaves space for difficult conversations, the kind that are necessary but easily avoided amid the daily-ness of life.

"Can we talk about the TACKLING PAIN project?" I ask. Simon hums an assent as he sets up the backgammon board.

We've maintained a minimal commitment to the project over the past few months. Every day, Simon has scribbled a journal entry over his morning coffee. And I too have established a consistent early morning routine of reading up on the current pain science literature, filling my notebooks with various facts, figures, and quotes. I paid the membership fees for us to join the International Association for the Study of Pain and the Canadian Pain Society. Since 1973, the IASP has been the leading global organization supporting the study of pain and the practice of pain relief. The Canadian Pain Society is our national chapter of the IASP. Becoming members allows Simon and me to access medical journals as well as in-person and online educational events. We both agree it's a solid start. Still, two months have passed and we have yet to build a sense of forward momentum or clear direction. I want to figure out why.

Part of the reason is obvious: we've been busy. Simon's August gig was quickly followed by another, then another. Despite my intention to take time off, shaky finances forced me to book extra days teaching Pilates. A month passed, then another, in a blur of responsible to-do lists. But I've begun to suspect that there are other, more subterranean reasons blocking our forward progression.

"We're not doing so great," I say.

"No," Simon agrees. "I guess not."

"We haven't compared notes in a while. Could we commit to a regular sit-down? A weekly TACKLING PAIN talk?"

Simon nods. "How about every Wednesday? A breakfast date?"

"That's good," I say. "Keep us accountable; keep us on track." I confess my suspicion that the IASP membership—while hugely valuable—also presented an enticing way to distract myself. Reading up on various theories of why some pain becomes chronic and some doesn't initially made me feel like I was doing something. Something important.

Something that might lead to something. But I had reached an impasse. The research studies were, by design, meant to analyze broad averages, not deal with individual outcomes. Yet, for us, the individual was everything. Within those mean averages, each percentage point represented a real person who, like Simon, was navigating life with a chronic condition, within their own unique context. Often the very design of the studies seemed to negate this quintessential aspect of the pain experience: that it was highly individualized. How truly helpful, then, could they be for me and Simon? In these articles pain was viewed as an abstract problem, an equation that hadn't quite been solved. A deep chasm existed between the puzzle-of-pain presented in these academic texts and the visceral force that exerted so much influence over both of our lives.

"Beau, I feel terrible thinking this," I say. "But in so many ways, I prefer the tidiness of the world of research to the messiness of life. I'll take averaged-pain-on-paper any day over individual-pain-screaming-beside-me-in-bed-in-the-middle-of-the-night."

"I get it," he says. "You and everyone else."

Simon faced his own quandary: talking, thinking, or journaling about pain when he was experiencing it was impossibly difficult. And, for the brief hours of respite in his day when the pain was more or less bearable? The last thing he wanted to do was talk, think, or journal about it.

"I'll be honest," he tells me now. "Sometimes you just mentioning the topic, or me thinking about journaling, will set it off."

So. These first few months have been disheartening. Despite our best intentions, our fragile agreement so far has only pitilessly underscored the fact that neither of us knows what to do, and so we distract ourselves as best we can, the bright potential of each morning replaced by the day's descending sense of never, ever doing enough to address the problem. Maybe the fact that we are now explicitly expressing that sentiment demonstrates progress, of a sort, but if so, it simply isn't enough.

"When we started, I wrote down a list of our key resources," I say, turning to the entry in my journal. "The main three being—one, our individual expressive abilities: you as a musician, me as a writer. Two, that we have each other. And Eli, and Chico, and the rest of the family, of course. And three, that we already have a pretty sophisticated understanding of the biology of pain."

"Okay, that's good," Si says. "But I'd add one more thing to your list of quest superpowers: we both have a long view of the healing process. I know, with pain, I want it to go away. Like, right now. But I also remember when I was in rehab, discouraged at how impossibly slowly things were progressing, you said that we shouldn't look at healing as being linear. That it was more of a spiral."

"I said that?"

"Impressive, right?" Si laughs. "But, really, it stuck with me."

"Okay, what do we say: *long view of spiral healing*?" Simon nods and I scribble it in the margin of the journal. "So next we need to identify our seemingly insurmountable obstacles. Every quest has a series of seemingly insurmountable obstacles."

"Well," Si says, "that's easy."

For the next twenty minutes, I transcribe furiously as Simon brainstorms the key obstacles to addressing his pain. The first is obvious: the pain itself.

Chronic pain is often described as being pain that lasts for more than three months, a definition so woefully incomplete that it is more misleading than helpful. One of the key factors that differentiates chronic pain from acute pain is its neuroplastic component. Over time the nervous system of the person-in-pain becomes increasingly adept at processing danger signals, thus creating an ongoing state of heightened sensitivity.

All of us have a strong passing familiarity with this concept of nervous system sensitization. For example, with a bout of the flu you might experience achy muscles, a dull headache, or sore eyes. Old injuries might flare up; sounds might boom louder or lights beam brighter. You might feel unexpectedly disheartened, pessimistic thoughts tumbling through your brain like damp clothes in an unending dryer cycle. Or perhaps you become alarmed by the suddenness and severity of the symptoms. Is this a regular flu? Or a new, potentially deadly, strain? Crawling into bed, you're empty of any thought except for this: *Every. Little. Thing. Hurts.*

Now imagine that in twenty-four hours the flu passes, but that "everything hurts" feeling doesn't go away. It lasts the week, then the month, then the season. Then years. Time dissolves as days blur together. That's chronic pain similar to the way Simon experiences it, and it's a major roadblock to doing anything at all.

When pain like this establishes itself, the second major obstacle becomes, well, everything else. Life. Good stress, stress that promotes growth and learning, no longer exists. Now all stress is too much. All stress is toxic fuel tossed onto the fire that is pain.

The founder of the field of stress research, Hans Selye, grounded his work primarily in a bodily understanding of the term—that is, stress as the result of injury, infection, or illness. But Simon and I primarily understand stress as a psychological process, as in: **blank** (work, kids, parents, partners, broken-down cars, accumulating bills, unfiled taxes, traffic, the global climate crisis, etc.) *is stressing me out*. Generally, this understanding of stress as a psychological process has come to dominate not just our cultural perception but also research. Ronald Melzack, one of the great innovators in pain research, challenged this perspective by insisting that it is critical to understand stress as "a biological system activated by physical injury, infection or any threat to biological homeostasis *as well as* by psychological threat." Both definitions, Melzack contended, are correct and important.

To avoid the ambiguities associated with the word *stress*, pain researchers generally prefer the term *allostatic load*. "Allostasis refers to the adaptive processes that maintain homeostasis through the production of mediators such as adrenalin, cortisol and other chemical messengers," researcher Bruce McEwen writes. "These mediators of the stress response promote adaptation in the aftermath of acute stress, but they also contribute to allostatic overload, the wear and tear on the body and brain that result from being 'stressed out.'" Excessive allostatic load is a key factor that contributes to pain; being pushed into a chronic state of allostatic *over*load can cause that pain to become increasingly persistent. Basically, if our problems (whether they be physical, psychological, or social) outweigh our ability to cope, it will likely result in some form of anguish, illness, or pain. We fall apart and—here's the kicker—in falling apart, our capacity for dealing with those problems is decreased further. Our coping resources become dangerously depleted.

As Simon says: "There's no gas in the tank. I'm running on empty."

It's not unusual for anxiety, stress, and pain states to be intimately connected, mutually reinforcing conditions that tend to aggravate one another. People who suffer from posttraumatic stress disorder are more likely to experience chronic pain at some point in life, and the reverse is also true. While numbers in the research fluctuate depending on variables (what kind of trauma was suffered; what kind of pain is being experienced), a conservative estimate suggests that people who experience chronic musculoskeletal pain are four times more likely to develop a diagnosable anxiety disorder. The list of allostatic factors that contribute to anxiety and/or pain will be different for everyone. For some, it might be an underlying health condition, repetitive strain from a demanding physical job, a specific genetic profile, or a history of trauma. For others, it might also include the daily experience of systemic racism or precarious income and housing.

The threshold for dealing with allostatic load will be different for everyone, but we all have our tipping point. A perfect storm of conditions exists for each of us that, no matter how resilient we are, will stress our nervous system beyond its capacity to cope. For Simon, that perfect storm came after navigating a year in which he barely survived a traumatic accident, then had to acclimatize to life in a wheelchair and reckon with a rapidly changing sense of self and role in the world. When the pain transformed on that fateful Thanksgiving weekend in 2009, he was in the midst of a potentially life-threatening MRSA infection. His immune system was under attack, he was routinely hospitalized, and discussions of amputating his infected foot became commonplace. I was his main support person, but I had reached my own state of crisis from prolonged stress. The world for both of us, but especially for him, was a very fragile place. Some of those stressors eventually receded, but Simon's nervous system, pushed past its tipping point, hasn't been able to fully bounce back.

A short list of his current allostatic factors would still include the physical trauma he survived, the continuing health implications of his injuries, and, finally, pain itself, along with the restrictions and isolation it continues to impose. Over the past month two interrelated factors have increased that allostatic load. First, there was a gig with slightly higher-than-usual stakes—the inaugural show of Simon's new band, Farm Team, where he debuted an entire set list of original songs. Second, an intense urinary tract infection flared up, requiring a daylong visit to our local ER. UTIs are a ubiquitous side effect of having a neurogenic bladder ("neurogenic" referring to the organ dysfunction that often accompanies brain, spinal cord, or nerve damage), a reality Simon has been contending with since his accident, but over the past year the infections had been both more persistent and more serious, resistant to a range of antibiotics.

Consequently, his nervous system, so sensitized by the biological stressors of pain and infection, was profoundly rattled by what used to be a normal and acceptable state of pre-gig jitters. The stress of the upcoming show massively disrupted his sleep patterns. Less sleep equaled more pain equaled more worry equaled less sleep equaled more pain, and so on and so on, creating the snake-eating-its-own-tail ouroboros of allostatic overload and chronic pain.

Over the past decade, we had dealt with UTIs by following a pragmatic routine for diagnosis and treatment. We couldn't stress too much over their presence—these types of infection were simply a fact of our new life. Best to, as Simon likes to say, suck it up, buttercup. Just deal with it. As far as strategies go, it was a pretty good one. Right up until the time... it wasn't.

"The UTIs have gotten so bad over the past year," I say. The candlelight throws flickering shadows across Simon's face as he nods in agreement. "It's a fine line between, on the one hand, being unfussy and proactive and, on the other, normalizing something that really shouldn't be normal. We've reached that point."

"Yeah," Si says. "We need to deal with the UTIs before we can move on to anything else. Can you write that down?" After I have done so, he takes the pen and adds an emphatic asterisk and three underlines.

But how to address it? Over the years, we've tried everything: countless antibiotic scripts and supplemental tonics; multiple procedures and significant diet changes. All to no avail. It was disheartening to work so hard at solving a problem and see so few results. Our sense of defeat grew exponentially with the build-up of failed attempts. And if this was true of UTIs, it was doubly true of pain. Since the pain first hit, Simon's moment-by-moment strategy has been to ignore it, to not, as he says, *give it any air time,* but that short-term outlook in no way represented the big picture over the past ten years. We had, in fact, expended a colossal amount of time, energy, and money attempting to address it directly.

After years of rotating physicians, we finally developed a stable relationship with kindly Dr. Jaschinski, and a specialist rehab doctor, our beloved Dr. Wilms, and both supported us in thinking inside and outside of the box in terms of pain management. We booked Feldenkrais, massage, craniosacral therapy, physiotherapy, acupuncture, and intramuscular stimulation sessions. Simon underwent several nerve block procedures. An occupational therapist recommended ways to make his wheelchair and computer work space more ergonomic, and on a physiotherapist's suggestion, Simon diligently used a TENS machine for two years, right up until the time the little electrical zaps started to increase his pain flares. A series of visits to a psychologist were enjoyable but time-consuming, the potential benefit, according to both Simon and the psychologist, not warranting the effort. With some creative financing, we installed an accessible swim spa unit (slightly bigger than a hot tub; much smaller than a pool) on our back patio, where Simon could either sit and relax in the jets or swim in place against a light current. It didn't reduce his pain, but it was one of the few fun and relaxing activities available to him.

Simon's accident had occurred at work, so there was financial support from WorkSafeBC (our provincial worker's compensation board) for some of these interventions. For others, we paid out of pocket. All of them exacted a high cost from our available time and energy. Together we shared a fantasy of a multidisciplinary rehab, or post-rehab, facility, a mythic place where people could go to be treated as whole persons and not just as atomized body parts, shuffled around from one specialist to another. It would be a nurturing kind of place, one that would acknowledge that the scope of chronic pain—or any kind of chronic illness—extends through all levels of an individual's existence, from the molecular all the way to the social. There, concurrent multimodal interventions would rebuild the energy of the suffering person, not dangerously deplete it.

Others have had a similar dream. John Bonica, the wrestler-turned-anesthesiologist and founder of the International Association for the Study of Pain, worked, from the 1950s on, to establish multidisciplinary pain management clinics in the U.S. The type of program he envisioned proved to be both effective and cost efficient, yet multidisciplinary clinics are still not a widely available option. In Canada, most programs operate in urban centers; the wait time for an initial consultation is five to six months on average, but it can be as long as five years—an eternity to a person-in-pain. We had discussed with Si's rehab doctor the possibility of getting him on a waitlist but eventually dismissed the idea. The type of pain clinic available to him was extremely limited in what it could offer, and, the doctor thought, it didn't warrant the disruption of relocating to a city for the duration of, say, a six-week program.

So, for now, the kind of healing center that Simon and I envision remains a pleasant but remote fantasy. Therapeutic interventions have happened in isolation, a fragmented approach that has never yielded a serious reduction in Simon's pain. But despite the fragmentation, we have really worked at it. This, then, is what we now identify as our third-biggest obstacle in the TACKLING PAIN project: What do you do when you have already tried everything?

"Well, not *everything*," Simon says. "I haven't been to a faith healer. Or a hypnotherapist."

"You scoff," I say. "But some of the most revolutionary pain scientists have not ruled out hypnotherapy."

"Are you suggesting that's where we start?"

"No—"

"Good, because I'm not rushing to book that appointment."

"No—" I'm interrupted again, this time by the hum of

returning power that momentarily animates the house—the fridge bristles, the heat pump purrs, and the overhead lights sputter on—then the hum falls silent and we're returned to darkness. Simon looks at me over the dancing candlelight, and sighs.

"So what next?"

That's the question, always the question. Early on, the idea that Simon's pain would persist was inconceivable to both of us. Surely there had to be a pill, or a procedure—some divine medical intervention—that would cure it. After each failed attempt, we would focus again, sighting our crosshairs on whatever that next thing would be that would solve the problem. But fighting pain is like shooting at shadows. Stuck in a state of perpetual twilight, it's difficult to see what comes next.

While I've stopped believing that there will be any easy answers or magical cures, I *do* still believe that with the right support, Simon himself can effect incremental changes in the quantity and quality of his pain. But, as Simon has often pointed out, there is a ruthlessness inherent to my position. For him, it feels about as useful, and compassionate, as a lifeguard telling someone who's drowning that now would be a good time to learn how to swim.

"But," Simon says, "swimming is one of my strengths. I've always been a good swimmer. Still, I don't know what to *do*."

"Yeah, well, if our three main obstacles to addressing pain are pain itself, life, and an utter lack of viable treatment options, it's hard to know where to go from there," I say. "Really all we can do is make—"

"—a to-do list. Oh, Stanley, you are so predictable."

"Not a to-do list. An *action plan*. Say, five short-term steps?"

"Okay. I'm listening."

"Well, on the one hand, I think we need to let go of the idea that a single solution exists. That some specialist, or some pill, or some procedure will provide an easy answer. We need to get curious. Focus on what *we* can do," I say.

"Okay, sure," Si says. "But, for the record, we've come to that realization multiple times over the last ten years. Personally I would prefer a magical medical cure. But—I can try again."

"Good. Then, on the other hand, we need help. Especially with the UTIs. Let's book an appointment with Dr. Wilms."

"That's a good step two."

"Next, we need to regularly continue these kinds of conversations. The difficult kind. The ones where we directly discuss the impact pain is having on both of us."

"What was the catchphrase you read me the other day: *pain denied is pain amplified*?"

"Exactly. It's the idea that when we deny or avoid facing pain—when we don't give ourselves the chance to move through it—we actually increase suffering."

"So step three: confront pain."

"Right, but also, step four, we need to stop focusing on stopping the pain. Paying no attention to pain might increase suffering, but so does paying *too* much attention."

"Okay, Goldilocks. So how do we find the *just right* amount of attention?"

"Well, my thought is, instead of trying to stop the negative thing—pain—we focus more on positives. Things that promote better health for you."

"Hmmm, all right. And step five?"

"I don't have a step five yet."

"Let me get this straight: you are suggesting that we, one, stop looking for outside solutions, and two, get some help?"

"Ahhh, yeah."

"Then, three, we directly confront pain, and four, we stop focusing so much on it."

"Yep. That about sums it up."

"Well, that's straightforward and not contradictory at all."

Once again, the house hums with electrical power, this time with more conviction. Sudden light brightens the room's dark corners, and Simon snuffs out the candle's wavering flame between his thumb and forefinger.

"Emerson said that foolish consistency was the hobgoblin of little minds," I say. "Oscar Wilde viewed it as a mark of the unimaginative. Huxley said the only truly consistent people were the dead."

"Geez, Stanley, did you memorize a whole page of Goodreads quotes? Also, you are the most consistent person I've ever known."

"Ouch."

"Well, consistently inconsistent, at least."

"That, I think, is my point about pain: consistently inconsistent."

"Right. Predictably unpredictable. That doesn't give me a lot to work with."

"No."

"But now the power is back on and I'd like to take a stab at addressing step four: stop focusing so much on pain and instead focus on improving overall health. Specifically, I would like to tackle this in the moment by ending this conversation, pumping up the heat, brewing a pot of tea, eating oatmeal cookies, and watching a Raptors game. Yeah? You with me?"

"That," I say, "sounds like a good start."

# 4

# Psykhē Sōmatikos

OCTOBER 10, DAY 80.

Simon hands me his journal at the outset of our breakfast date and I read his morning entry:

> *I wake to that nagging, jangling alarm clock inside my body. It robs me of the focus needed to get real work done and it leaves me reeling to start the day. If I must live with this pain, it would be great if it was useful in an artistic sense, but it never delivers a melody, this raging muse. Maybe I need to score the pain, write a symphony or lyrics set to Beethoven's Fifth (something like* get me some new drugs, ow ow ow ow*). But every lyrical invention I come up with seems to be a variation of a whiny "I'm trying, I'm trying, I'm really really trying"... then I run out of steam.*

"It's rough to read, Beau," I say. Common themes have emerged in his journal entries: he feels unfocused, out of sync, alone, dangerously tired. "One of your greatest strengths, I think, is your ability to connect with people. And your energy."

"That comes from being a musician," Si says. "From practicing the art of good dynamic timing within a band. Playing in the pocket. It used to, anyways. My innate sense of time now is about as musical and connected as two skeletons fucking on a tin roof."

"Colorful image."

He laughs. "Years ago, a hip bassist described a dysfunctional rhythm section that way to me. I've waited a long time to use it in a proper context."

"Well done," I say. "Do you think the journaling is helping?"

"It's good to have a spot where you can lay down unsayable thoughts, the ones you think and then immediately wish you hadn't," Si says. "And it limits complaining time. If I can get it all out in fifteen minutes in the morning, then, ideally, it frees up my mind for the rest of the day."

"You don't complain that much," I say.

"Well, good. I'm trying to write down more upbeat stuff too, because we all know it's best to have an attitude of gratitude. Of course, it's also important to leave a little latitude..." Simon grins into a lengthening pause and I sense a coming punchline: "... for baditude."

"Baditude—it's a good band name," I say. "What about adding a daily log of your pain scores to your journals? Then we can track the day-to-day over, say, three months."

This is not a new strategy for us: several times, in the aftermath of a procedure, Simon has been asked to track his pain for a few weeks. But the subjectivity of self-report is a perpetually thorny issue in the history of pain treatment. The standard *on a scale of one to ten how bad is your pain* question doesn't exactly yield a nuanced rating. Although more detail-oriented questionnaires do exist, as far as Simon and I are concerned, their existence is purely academic. In more than a decade of dealing with chronic pain, Simon has only ever been asked the basic one-to-ten question.

"No pain rating," Simon says. I am surprised by his outright rejection and say so.

"It's an irritating waste of time. Time I don't have to waste. Maybe for others it's instructive, but for me, it never feels very accurate. I'm always wading through a basic three-to-five level of pain, but the bad stuff comes in spikes. The seven-eight-nine-ten jolts. One afternoon I might get three isolated super-ten jolts and that's it. Another day, I'm bombarded with an unending series of seven jolts. Which is worse? I don't know. They both suck, but 'suck' doesn't have a clear numerical value. It's not helpful. And it makes me grumpy."

"Okay," I say. "Personally, I see value in being able to observe long-term patterns, but, as you wish, we'll table tracking pain scores. Final thought: apps."

"Apps?"

"Yeah, there's a ton of them. Ones that track things like the severity of your symptoms and possible triggers, medications, activity level. Some have mindfulness meditation prompts or exercise suggestions or meal plans. That kind of thing."

For weeks, my online pain research had been bombarded with ads featuring a close-up of a woman, head in hands, the taut contours of her face holding a lonely howl within, while around her the world dissolves into a foggy blur. The face of pain. After about the tenth appearance of Our Lady of Sorrows, I clicked the link for CurableHealth.com. Curable's mission, the website informed me, is to "reach every person with chronic symptoms, and present them with the opportunity to improve their lives" through a commitment to making the latest advances in pain science understandable, convenient, and affordable.

"Affordable, hey? How much does it cost?" Simon asks.

"It's $4.99 a month to subscribe—"

"Ahh, financial death by a million and one $4.99 monthly subscriptions—"

"—but they're offering a seven-day free trial," I say, opening the page on his iPad.

We hunch over the screen at the kitchen table, getting acquainted with Clara, the app's virtual pain coach. The interface is a mix between a choose-your-own-adventure story and texting a friend. Clara sends a series of "texts," and then the user is given a choice of "text" replies. By asking these preset questions, Clara tailors the app to your unique pain profile. Clicking on certain texts activates Clara into speech, her manner engaging as she outlines aspects of pain biology. Can an app be genuine? Clara seems so. Her voice is young, friendly, smart: attractive in a bookish but athletic way. The kind of person who bikes to work, wears her flaxen hair in an unfussy ponytail, and hikes on the weekend with her goofy goldendoodle, Chester. She wants to have kids one day, but not right now.

Simon is attentive as he navigates through the cautions and various questions:

*If at any time you feel unable to manage your emotions or feel out of control, contact a licensed professional.*

*Do you really want to believe this can work for you?*

*Do you really want to believe you could be in less pain a month from now? And a month from then, you might not have any pain at all?*

"Do I *want* to *believe?*" Simon says. "Clara's starting to sound like a faith healer."

"And, obviously, if Curable's program doesn't work for you in a month or two, it's not their fault. You just didn't *want* to *believe* it enough," I say.

"Ha!" Simon continues to scroll, choosing a four-minute sound bite on the role the amygdala plays in pain processing. "Cool," he says when it's completed, then taps back to the main screen.

After a few more friendly, inquisitive pseudo-texts, the interface offers a list of options. Simon clicks on a link titled "Perfectionism."

"Why 'Perfectionism'?" I ask. "I don't know anyone who excels more at the boy's art of why-work-hard-for-an-A+-when-a B-will-do-just-fine."

"Harsh," Simon says. "But fair. No, I'm clicking on this for you, my chronically overextended friend. You've never really understood the importance of strategic laziness."

Clara, in her measured and mellifluous tone, explains that perfectionism is, in our high-performance culture, a useful and valued trait. However, it is a way of being in the world that extracts a high cost.

Perfectionists experience a continuous sense of urgency to do more and to do better. Tension builds, allostatic load increases, and this affects emotional and physical resilience. When the demands perfectionists make of themselves exceed their functional ability, tipping them into allostatic *overload*, they experience a state of high anxiety, which leaves a tangible imprint in the body—heart rate rises, stress hormones are released, and the fight-or-flight response amps up—a kind of self-perpetuating physiological emergency mode. The wound-up nervous system of a perfectionist is, in fact, predisposed to amplify pain.

The antithesis of the perfectionist's habitual anxiety is an outlook of relaxed awareness where one is capable of experiencing joy and gratitude, or an immersion in and acceptance of the present moment. These experiences, too, have an effect on the body, releasing chemicals that can potentially reduce pain. Yet, Clara explains, perfectionists rarely indulge in the kind of spontaneous play that leads to these grace states, and so they move through life accumulating a surplus of high-anxiety, pain-amplifying moments and a deficiency of calming, restorative ones.

What can the poor perfectionist do? Well, awareness that there is a downside to being a high achiever is an important first step to finding better balance between work and play. Perfectionists need to practice being kind to themselves. Clara suggests holding yourself to a standard you would hold a good friend to, someone who you want to excel but in a healthy, well-rounded way.

"Hmmm," Simon says.

"Hmmm," I say.

"Half hour is up. Goodbye, Clara. You've given me something to think about." He powers down the iPad. "But as a lifelong anti-perfectionist, and current chronic pain sufferer, it's now time for me to take a nap."

AS THE DAY WEARS ON I find myself inexplicably irritated by the Curable app's concept of perfectionism as it relates to persistent pain, even though the idea that the perfectionist's worldview might affect their physiological resilience makes sense to me. As Simon cheekily noted, I've struggled with managing high anxiety since childhood. In fact, if Clara had taken a snapshot of Simon and me at twenty-five—Kara, an introverted, self-conscious worrier and Simon, a gregarious, spontaneous extrovert—clearly all bets would be on me to be the one to suffer chronic pain later in life.

Is the concept of perfectionism relevant to Simon at all? One of the consequences of Simon's injuries is that he now experiences more anxiety. Initially this stress centered on the unpredictability of his neurogenic bowel and bladder. The possibility of incontinence is always present, and for years he has tortured himself trying to find the precise combination of actions, medications, and foods to ensure that his bowels behave. Given the damaged wiring of his nervous system, his efforts don't always work.

Could the anxiety of this daily stressor have introduced Simon to a mindset that, while not exactly perfectionism, is, let's say, perfectionism-adjacent? It seems a reasonable proposition. To make matters worse, the pain itself magnifies this stress. When the mild electric current that troubled Simon's hips and low back transformed into neuropathic bolts of lightning, the world became much less safe, and Simon's normal confident approach was replaced with a state of constant, fretful vigilance. What if the pain hits, Simon now asks himself, while I'm in the middle of a gig? While I'm driving? Teaching a guitar lesson? Eating dinner with friends? As controlling for these variables becomes less possible, he is more inclined to limit those activities.

This, it seems to me, is how the concept of perfectionism is relevant to Simon's situation. The opposite of pain is not so much pleasure as it is vigor, wonder, curiosity. What the person-in-pain loses over time is a sense of ease in their environment. Like the perfectionist, the person-in-pain experiences a surplus of high-anxiety, pain-amplifying moments and a deficiency of calming, restorative ones. This, then, is the source of my irritation: it's not just the Curable app but the world at large that tends to apply one-dimensional labels, like "perfectionist," to a person-in-pain without necessarily accounting for the nuances of such a complex experience. Like, for example, the fact that the perfectionist's stress and desperate need to control the uncontrollable might not necessarily be a mindset that precedes chronic pain but instead might be a by-product of that pain.

Is this a necessary distinction to make?

The answer, for me, is a resolute yes. But why?

It is, I realize as I move through my afternoon chores, because I'd like to shield Simon from the kinds of characterizations and labels the world pins on a pain sufferer. And at the root of this defensive response is a man named René.

RENÉ DESCARTES, THE MAN who coined *Cogito, ergo sum*, or *I think, therefore I am*, hands-down the catchiest phrase of the seventeenth century, is largely responsible for establishing the post-Enlightenment template for thinking about mind, body, and pain. In 1664, Descartes published the *Treatise on Man*, which included the infamous drawing of a chubby man-boy kneeling, his front foot in perilous proximity to the billowing flames of an open campfire. In Descartes's conceptualization, a long, hollow tube, like a thin hose, travels from the reckless boy's foot all the way to his brain. Inside the tube is an activating substance similar, Descartes thought, to a "fine wind" or a "lively flame," which he named "animal spirits." The animated tube acts as a kind of cord that is tugged when encountering unpleasant or dangerous stimuli (like an open fire), ringing an alarm bell inside the brain. Animal spirits are alerted, and it's their action that causes our man-boy to pull his stinging toes back from the fire. *Ouch*. Et voilà! Pain. It's a simple picture that reinforces our most common experiences of acute (or nociceptive) pain, and one that formed the current foundation of medical science's conceptualization of a pain-state.

Descartes was the great-great grandpapa of the mind-body split, also known as Cartesian dualism, the kind of either-or, black-or-white binary thinking that has influenced the last four hundred years of Western thought. The thinking mind, according to Descartes, was distinct from, and placed above, all other forms of material life. Unfortunately for us, as the cultural inheritors of Cartesian dualism, it is a profoundly limited cosmology that in its insistence to divide the Self from the Other has ruptured an individual sense of biological interconnectedness.

But pain, and its various complexities, has always been the wrench tossed into the mechanistic Cartesian worldview. This was true even for Descartes, who in 1641 wrote:

> Nature teaches me by these sensations of pain... that I am not only lodged in my body as a pilot in a vessel, but that I am very closely united to it, and so to speak so intermingled with it that I seem to compose one whole... For all these sensations of hunger, thirst, pain etc. are in truth none other than certain confused modes of thought which are produced by the union and apparent intermingling of body and mind.

It's hard to understand how dualism gained such a strong foothold in our collective consciousness given the fact that, when it came to pain, Descartes himself was obviously not a paragon of consistency. While his intellectual endeavors helped kick off the Enlightenment, or the Age of Reason, it would have been impossible for him to foresee the groundswell of colonialist cultural, scientific, and geopolitical change he helped initiate, or how the developing profession of medicine would eagerly embrace the notion of the mind-body split for the way in which it offered a clearly defined arena of expertise. Now the concrete, mechanical world of the body irrefutably belonged to men of science while troubling questions of the mind, spirit, or soul were best left to the musings of theologians, philosophers, wise women, and artists.

The invention of the microscope in the late sixteenth century was followed by the development of more and more powerful diagnostic aids: stethoscopes, ophthalmoscopes, X-rays, MRIs. Powerful tools, certainly, that have helped us understand, and rescue, the human body in profound and astounding ways. But, as the medical historian Roy Porter has pointed out, these new technologies also transformed medicine from a practice where doctors asked a patient *What is the matter?* to one where the central question has become *Where does it hurt?* In the four hundred years post-Descartes, the power dynamic shifted irrefutably from patients, and their accounts of ailments, to physicians and their all-powerful, all-seeing machines.

This brisk progression of science and technology occurred alongside equally rapid cultural change. Literacy and education spread, clearly defined professions and bureaucracies were developed, and capitalist economies expanded, all changes that both increased and thrived on social stability. The ideal citizen was energetic, self-sufficient, entrepreneurial, and, above all else, healthy. But as profit-making became the dominant organizing principle of social life, the world also grew more inhospitable to any person not able to fully embody these qualities of rugged individualism. Vulnerable people—the elderly, the disabled, the ill, or anyone, really, navigating a short- or long-term phase of dependency—were pushed to the margins of society.

Pain, in this new world order, was an octagonal peg roughly shoved into a round hole. Its mind-shattering extremes combined with its radical subjectivity provoked intense cultural anxiety. Often, there was no definitive proof of pain, no way to adequately measure or quantify its existence, which had to rely instead upon the self-report of the sufferer. This was especially problematic if the person-in-pain required time off from work, or worse, social aid in the form of financial assistance. When profit-making trumps caregiving, any plea for help is viewed in a dubious light. Pain, along with disability, becomes inherently suspicious. "To have great pain is to have certainty," Elaine Scarry famously wrote in *The Body in Pain,* "to hear that another person has pain is to have doubt."

We can't blame it all on Descartes, a man who valued mind above all else, for it is history's trajectory that neatly inverted his dichotomy into new, more bureaucratically functional hierarchies: acute pain was more creditable than chronic; detectable physical pains more valid than elusive, invisible ones. As a social framework for advancing our understanding of pain, dualistic thinking has been egregiously inadequate and punitive to a great many suffering people. And, despite cultural pushback, it still exerts significant influence.

Evidence of dualism's pernicious sway in the world of health and wellness can be seen in the abundance of self-help titles that refer to the mind-body connection, a syntactical construction that presumes a potential state of disconnect, a rift that continually needs to be bridged. But one of the tough lessons we learned in the wake of Simon's accident and in the face of his pain is that every injury, or illness, will have an accompanying set of emotions, thoughts, beliefs, and memories that will influence the impact of that injury or illness. And all mental anguish, such as intense terror, grief, or anxiety, leaves its traces in the tissues of the body, altering muscle tension, the production of stress hormones, and the body's ability, at a cellular level, to heal. The thinking mind and the moving body might be in a state of dysfunction, but they are never separate, or disconnected. All things mind-body constitute a borderless blending, a two-way dance either in or out of harmony.

Still, neither Simon nor I are completely immune from the influence of dualism. Even though we reject the notion of a mind-body split, the uncomfortable truth is, when his pain began, both of us immediately took comfort in the knowledge that it was directly related to the intense trauma he survived. It was physical, not psychological. It was not psychosomatic; it was *real.*

This opposition of *real* and *psychosomatic* is deeply ingrained in our cultural thinking. But the etymology of "psychosomatic" is from the Greek: *psykhē* meaning "mind"; *sōmatikos* meaning "body." From roughly 1938 on, it has been used to describe physical disorders that spring from psychological causes, with a generally pejorative sense of cuckoo flimflammery. Etymologically, though, there is no reason the term could not as easily apply in reverse, describing emotional disorders that derive from physical causes.

Given this definition, it could be argued that there is nothing in the realm of human existence that *isn't* psychosomatic.

People-in-pain are acutely aware of the potential labels that attend their condition: as patients, they are time-consuming, problematic, noncompliant. Certain pain clinics boast that they cater to patients that have *failed all other interventions.* Why, I wonder, is it that the patient has failed, and not the interventions? Why make pain treatment a pass-or-fail process? Why must so many of the descriptors of people-in-pain be so inherently judgmental? Would it be so difficult to acknowledge that it is not the person-in-pain but rather the experience of pain that is time-consuming, problematic, frustratingly noncompliant?

Unfortunately, the self-help world of health and fitness is often equally judgmental, entrenched as it is in the colloquial belief that our personal outlook is *entirely* responsible for determining biological outcomes. As a Pilates and movement teacher, I bump into this attitude all the time. Cloaked in a sheen of dewy positivity, this approach at its best encourages people to bring awareness to their negative thought and behavior patterns and supports making changes to increase well-being. But at its worst, this perspective once again equates illness and pain with a kind of moral failing, strongly implying that if you're not getting better, then you're just not putting in the work to evolve your mind into a state of health. For a person-in-pain, this can be yet one more societal faction weighing in and pronouncing your very personhood as wanting: damaged, defective, unworthy.

"It's the brain-or-the-mind issue all over again," Si says after listening to my rant on the perils of stereotyping people-in-pain as perfectionists. He's up from his nap and has joined me in the kitchen for dinner prep.

"Right? People tend to want to reduce pain to an either-or construction. In the medical model, *real* pain is a symptom of an underlying problem in bodily tissues; in the everyday non-medical model, pain is all psychological, a problem of how we think and behave."

"Maybe," Si says as he sautés a pan of garlic and onions, "part of the difficulty in confronting pain springs from the deep divide between those two perspectives." He lays the spatula on the spoon-rest and looks up at me. "It's being stranded in that gap where people really suffer."

"Truth."

"And that's definitely me: lost in rogue territory."

"That," I say, adding a box of pasta to a boiling pot of water, "is insightful. I think this TACKLING PAIN project is starting to work."

Simon smiles. "Don't be smug. But you're right. I've definitely just had my first aha! moment."

# 5

# Welcoming the Unwelcome

OCTOBER 11, DAY 81.

Over the next week, Simon and I commit to exploring what we have now dubbed rogue territory.

"Potentially fertile. Definitely uncharted," Simon says. "It's a place where songs might live."

"That's good," I say.

"I don't know if it's good, exactly," he says. "But at least it's something."

Our plan is for Simon to focus on the Curable app to maximize the free trial while I do a research dive into the work of a well-known name in the pain industry: Dr. John Sarno.

Sarno was an early, and controversial, pioneer in attempting to bridge the gap between the physical and the psychological. During his heyday, in the 1980s and '90s, he was either derided or ignored by his medical peers, and yet he amassed a devoted following of patients. A physician who notoriously eschewed the traditional peer-reviewed research process, Sarno developed his insights through his practical experience of treating patients, and in this he was prolific: thousands claimed they had recovered from chronic low back pain using his methods.

In many ways, Sarno was ahead of his time. Despite a pervasive lack of research to support his position, he insisted on the emotional component of pain, recognizing that overly fearful or catastrophizing thoughts were bound to make things worse. And in the 1980s, when bed rest was the accepted prescription for back pain, Sarno, ever the contrarian, was a fierce advocate of resuming physical activity as soon as possible. He was also dismissive of a reliance on scans, noting that many of the common findings on X-rays or MRIs were "normal abnormalities" and didn't accurately represent clear-cut causes for continuing pain. These insights, which were considered radical—or downright wacky—at the end of the twentieth century are now, twenty years later, backed by a growing body of research.

Sarno's belief was that nearly all chronic pain was caused by repressed emotions, or what Freud referred to as somatic conversions: the process by which the crafty unconscious mind translated deep personal conflict into bodily symptoms. Sarno hypothesized that the brain created pain by reducing blood flow to various parts of the body—neck, shoulders, back, tush—as an elaborate means of distraction, enabling a person to avoid facing up to their messiest emotions. Do you constantly feel like an imposter? Do you feel unhappy and powerless at work? Or, perhaps—and this, in keeping with Sarno's Freudian roots, was a common theme—you have unresolved issues with your parents? This pain-process, which he labeled tension myositis syndrome, could be cured through psychotherapy, or journaling, or a combination of both, as a way to confront the uncomfortable emotions wreaking so much havoc in the body. If you could exorcise all your subconscious negativity through the act of daily expressive writing, you could be freed of physical pain.

There is an evangelical quality to the testimonials of Sarno's patients that Simon and I find wildly irritating, though it's not because we don't agree that fearful or catastrophizing thoughts tend to make any situation worse. And Sarno's key interventions—confront the difficult or repressed, rebuild the good, find the help needed to empower yourself to take control of your own pain management—are uncannily like the action plan Simon and I have constructed. It's more the reductive nature of the patient claims that get our hackles up. *All* chronic pain cannot be boiled down to a manifestation of repressed rage or an enduring conflict with your mother—equations many Sarno acolytes tend to insist upon. Displaced emotional distress might be the root cause of bodily pain for some, even for many—but not for all, and an insistent, generalized application of Sarno's theories diminishes their overall credibility.

Still, Sarno's message continues to resonate, even after his death in 2017; judging by the websites devoted to promoting his vision and the vast number of self-help books urging chronic pain sufferers to confront the unpleasant emotions underlying their pain, it promises to endure.

"Maybe John Sarno is like aspirin," I say, as Simon and I clear away our breakfast dishes. Leaves and bark containing salicylic acid have been used since around 3000 BCE for fevers and pain. And in 1899, the German pharmaceutical company Bayer created the synthetic compound acetylsalicylic acid, naming their new wonder drug "aspirin." But no one could explain, exactly, *how* aspirin worked until the 1970s, when the British pharmacologist John

Vane published research for which he was later awarded a Nobel Prize.

"So what you're saying is that while we don't yet understand *how* Sarno's methods work for so many people, we just know they do." Simon starts the dishwasher. "Does anybody know? I mean, other doctors must have picked up where he left off."

"It's a good question. That's going to be my focus this week while you mess around with Curable."

"Deal." Simon fist-bumps me as he heads to his office.

CURABLE'S SCIENTIFIC ADVISORY BOARD is an impressive list of leading experts in pain research and treatment, several of whom are, in light of groundbreaking new scientific insights, currently updating Sarno's therapeutic legacy. I zero in on Les Aria, the Lead Pain Psychologist for the Kaiser Permanente Medical Group in Northern California. His Curable bio states that his practice incorporates elements of modern pain science, mindfulness, and acceptance and commitment therapy, the final line reading: *His passion for mind-body interventions promotes a unique style to help patients relate differently to their suffering, and thereby shift them into pain recovery and wellness.* It's a sentence that appeals to me, first, because he uses the verb *shift* instead of *cure,* a distinction that seems both realistic and honest. Second, I appreciate the phrase *pain recovery* for the way it hovers somewhere between the more typically heard phrases, *pain management* (defeatist right out of the gate) or *pain solution* (too much hubris). *Pain recovery* describes a dynamic, open-ended process, and I like that. I email Dr. Aria describing the project Simon and I have undertaken and ask if he would be willing to chat. Fifteen minutes later my inbox dings with a new message containing the welcoming subject line: HAPPY TO HELP.

"MY CAREER IS a good example of never say never," Dr. Aria says, laughing on the other end of the phone where I've reached him at home in Northern California. It's Saturday, early. A notorious rambler, I have made concise notes to direct my questions so as not to intrude too deeply into his personal downtime. But Dr. Aria is generous in his answers and our conversation relaxes into an easy, unrushed tempo.

He describes how a decades-spanning career treating persistent pain seemed an unlikely outcome the day when, during his medical residency, he began a clerkship in a chronic pain clinic. A patient, angry at being denied meds, flung a chair across the room. Dr. Aria, who was still in the process of figuring out the direction his career in medicine would take, remembers thinking clearly: *Not this. Anything but this.*

"So I returned to my training as a neuropsychologist," he explains. "I had a love affair with the brain, but that in turn led back to the issue of pain. I have loved mysteries ever since I was a kid, and pain is one of the biggest mysteries out there. I started to think that there were maybe better options available to treat this unique patient population."

Early in his career Dr. Aria was treating an elderly woman with extreme back pain. "I asked her: Besides your back, what else in your life is hurting?" It was a breakthrough moment. The woman described the extreme isolation she was experiencing. Her family was overseas, and she was disconnected and alone. The prospect of aging in this manner was overwhelming. Together they addressed the issue of her isolation, finding practical ways for her to reconnect with both family and community. When these emotional needs were met, her pain began to shift. Since then, Dr. Aria has gone on to treat over three thousand patients with an unusually good rate of pain resolution. "I would say approximately 80 percent of my patients reach a state of recovery."

Like Sarno, Dr. Aria has experienced being an outlier. Among many of his pain clinician peers, it's generally accepted that the best outcome for a chronic pain patient is a workable pain management strategy. Dr. Aria believes there is good reason to have more hope, although the lack of practitioners who share his philosophy has often left him feeling alone in his beliefs. But over the last five years, the science supporting his approach has grown much stronger, and he has connected with like-minded mavericks like Howard Schubiner, David Hanscom, and, perhaps most significantly, a soft-spoken researcher named Stephen Porges. "Finally, I've been able to quiet some of my own internal doubts," Dr. Aria explains. "I'm much more confident now in saying, this is how healing works."

For Dr. Aria, healing begins by acknowledging that pain in life is unavoidable. "But suffering is more like a mental script used to narrate that reality," he explains. "And this is where we all have a choice." The therapeutic process of intentionally examining, then rewriting, a narrative of suffering is both layered and dynamic. Dr. Aria begins with what he calls the three R's: re-educate, re-tune, and re-engage.

The first step, **re-educate**, begins with the same question Simon and I started out with: What is pain? Why do I hurt? Dr. Aria provides a primer of modern pain neuroscience for patients. "I always start with explaining that usually the issue is not really the tissue," Dr. Aria says. "Pain is always a product of the brain."

"Simon and I keep returning to that basic maxim, understanding it in new ways," I say. "Although Simon prefers the statement that pain is made by his nervous system. *Interpreted* by his nervous system."

"And that's brilliant," Dr. Aria says. "Because that's exactly what it is. Many persistent problems that present as musculoskeletal issues are really issues of the nervous system. A foundation in current science helps patients understand this."

It's this state of dysfunction that makes the next step of **re-tuning** the nervous system so complex. Dr. Aria begins with a ten-day schedule following something called the Safe and Sound Protocol. During the protocol, clients wear specially designed headphones to listen to algorithmically filtered music that stimulates the neural networks associated with listening, training the middle ear muscles to tune in to cues of safety signaled by the frequencies of the human voice.

Created by Stephen Porges, the Safe and Sound Protocol grew out of his groundbreaking work developing the Polyvagal Theory, or as it's sometimes called, "the science of feeling safe." Polyvagal Theory focuses on the critical role the tenth cranial nerve, also known as the vagus nerve, plays in regulating both our physiological and psychological health. The vagus is the longest nerve in the body, traveling in two directions: down to the lungs, heart, diaphragm, and stomach and up to the neck, throat, eyes, and ears. It's a literal bridge between mind and body, a thrumming internal power line of bi-directional communication that helps regulate things like heart rate, blood pressure, sweating, and digestion.

Porges coined the term "neuroception" to describe how the vagus nerve is constantly receiving feedback from the world outside and inside of us, assessing this ongoing flurry of threat and safety cues, and then determining an appropriate response. This lightning-fast process occurs in the primitive parts of the brain, generally without our conscious awareness, and it is expressed through three main physiological states: the relaxed, responsive parasympathetic state, where social connection and intimacy occur; the sympathetic state, where we react to a sense of danger with either a fight or flight response; and the frozen dorsal vagal state, in which the feeling of threat is so overwhelming we become immobilized. The Safe and Sound Protocol is designed to ease an overtaxed nervous system out of the latter two states and into the first, where, ideally, a person is more relaxed and socially available. It's been used to treat the distress experienced by children and adults with autism spectrum disorder, or those recovering from trauma or anxiety.

"I use Safe and Sound with a patient thirty minutes once a day for ten days, and it provides a kind of shortcut to addressing the physiological underpinnings of stress," Dr. Aria explains. "My pops was a naval officer and he had a saying: *no teaching through a storm*. Meaning it is almost impossibly difficult to learn something new when immersed in a state of emergency. Safe and Sound is a way to ease people out of the storm. It saves a lot of treatment time. After only ten days, patients feel more relaxed and receptive. Ready for the next phase of therapy."

Dr. Aria is trained in cognitive behavioral therapy (CBT), a psychotherapeutic approach that focuses on the relationships between thoughts, feelings, and actions and is used to address a variety of psychological and behavioral issues, like anxiety, depression, or obsessive-compulsive disorders. In a multidisciplinary approach, it's widely considered a cornerstone of effective chronic pain treatment, seeking to identify the negative thought patterns that contribute to, or even create, a pain-state and reframe them in a more positive light. More positive thoughts, CBT advocates contend, mean more positive emotions mean more positive behaviors. ("Let me get this straight," Si said when we discussed CBT earlier. "If Sisyphus could only stop complaining about how much his daily grind hurts or how heavy his boulder is, he might begin to see things in a different light?" "It's likely a little more nuanced," I said. "But, essentially, yeah. That's it.")

CBT, Dr. Aria explains now, provided him with a solid therapeutic foundation, but as his practice evolved, his focus shifted to an alternate approach: acceptance and commitment therapy (ACT). Incorporating many elements of CBT, ACT adds two more key ingredients to the therapeutic gumbo: a mindfulness practice and a "commitment to action" plan.

While there is overlap, CBT and ACT differ in their frameworks. The explicit aim of CBT interventions is to reduce or manage pain through the reframing of negative thought patterns; ACT, instead, focuses on cultivating a vital life while accepting that pain is a normal and inevitable sensation, and that many of the emotions associated with a pain-state, like fear or anxiety, are also normal and inevitable.

"One of the big differences between CBT and ACT," Dr. Aria tells me, "is that ACT makes room in the process to welcome the unwelcome. Observing some of our messier thoughts is the first step in being able to make active choices. Because only once you acknowledge *how* you are thinking can you ask: Is this working for me? Or is there a different approach I could take?"

It takes approximately eight to twelve weeks to work through an ACT program, which begins with clients bringing a focused, nonjudgmental awareness to multiple areas of their life. Next comes the tricky stage of, as Dr. Aria says, "opening up to what's showed up." This can be a difficult, emotional time, but it often leads to unexpected insights and breakthroughs which, in turn, promote a greater degree of self-knowledge. "I can help a client acquire the skills necessary to increase their psychological flexibility in twelve weeks. But as a practice, ACT is lifelong. And ultimately that's a commitment the client must make themselves. It's a very practical behavioral therapy for anybody," Dr. Aria explains. "Clients and clinicians alike."

The work done to re-educate and re-tune the nervous system lays the foundation for Dr. Aria's third and final R: **re-engagement**. Here, he supports a client to develop strategies that will help them re-engage in the activities and relationships they most value, but that they may have lost as they struggled with pain. Re-engaging often starts with gradually exposing yourself to the activity. Your ultimate goal might be to run a half-marathon, but you'd start with a daily ten-minute walk.

Dr. Aria's use of the Safe and Sound Protocol is a unique aspect of his practice, but one he hopes will become more commonplace. He's working with researchers at Indiana University to create the kind of peer-reviewed research necessary to make his colleagues pay attention.

"I think Safe and Sound would be helpful for Simon," I say.

"Complex pain syndromes like Simon's make up about 1 percent of my practice," Dr. Aria says. "When the pain is caused by injury to the nervous system itself, that's the most mysterious pain of all. I often use the analogy of malfunctioning wiring in a house. You switch on a light, and it activates the garbage disposal, or the upstairs toilet flushes. It can be very unpredictable." He pauses on the other end of the phone line before adding: "But the great thing about Safe and Sound is that there's no downside in terms of negative side effects, like there may be with meds or other interventions. Healing might be a longer, more complicated process for Simon than for many, but calming the nervous system is always going to be a good place to start."

SIMON AND I SIT DOWN to go over the notes of my conversation with Dr. Aria. We decide two things. While Simon thinks that following a twelve-week program would be helpful, we don't have easy access to one, and pursuing it will only tax our resources of time, energy, and money. Our homegrown action plan is sufficiently compatible with an ACT approach that we're going to keep forging ahead on our own. Second, we *do* want to follow up on the Safe and Sound Protocol. It's not a treatment option for Simon currently, but Dr. Aria has provided me with a link to Unyte, the company that has partnered with Stephen Porges to sell his Polyvagal

Theory–associated products. Simon and I browse the site and decide to purchase an iom2, a biofeedback device that offers an "interactive meditation program."

"Whatever that is," Simon says.

"You need to prepare yourself as we do a deep dive into neuroplastic pain treatments that the word *mindfulness* is going to come up. A lot," I say.

The concept of meditation has always been a hard sell for Simon, who also has a keen dislike for the word *mindfulness* and the way it's been degraded to meaninglessness through overuse and commercialization. As far as he's concerned, our uniquely narcissistic Western culture is guilty of extracting ancient practices from Buddhist texts and transforming them into a society-wide program of endless self-improvement. He has a point, even if it is a cynical one. But recently I've embarked on an unapologetic mindfulness propaganda campaign, reminding him how fundamental the concept is to all somatic practices—like the Alexander Technique, Pilates, or Feldenkrais—with the great Moshé Feldenkrais coining the phrase "Awareness Through Movement." Jon Kabat-Zinn, too, was pivotal in bringing the concept of mindfulness to Western culture through his Mindfulness-Based Stress Reduction program, a practice that is less spiritual and more common sense in nature. Kabat-Zinn defined mindfulness as simply being awareness that arises through paying attention, "on purpose, in the present moment, and non-judgmentally." But it's when I threaten to bombard Simon with research papers demonstrating the ways in which a mindfulness practice helps to reduce activity in the amygdala, the area of the brain central to the experience of fear—and how that reduction in activity interrupts a toxic pain-and-fear cycle, which in turn helps to reduce the experience of chronic pain—that he finally relents.

"It's going to be your own personalized mindfulness device," I say now, pointing at the screenshot of the iom2.

"Ew. Gross," Si says, laughing. "But, then again, according to my daily internet feed, I will soon be transformed into my very best self. All through my immaculate mindfulness. Get ready for the new Simon: I'll have a better mood and improved sleep and eating habits; I'll be a stronger person with enhanced leadership and athletic skills. Also, apparently, a better lover."

"Well, okay, then. The iom2 is definitely worth a hundred bucks."

"But what if I start posting pictures of sunsets and raindrops dripping off flower petals on Instagram, signing everything with a #livelaughlove?"

"Then I'll know I've created a monster."

Our second product choice is the Dreampad, a pillow that hooks up to your phone or iPad. Gentle vibrations accompany music being played through the pillow, triggering a relaxation response in the nervous system. It's not exactly the Safe and Sound Protocol, but it seems like the next best thing.

We place our order and get an estimated delivery date; a package should arrive in two weeks' time. We sit in my office momentarily basking in the novel sensation of making progress.

"Although all we've really done," Simon says, "is throw money at the pain problem. And are we certain that this is better than spending the money on cartons of Pralines 'n' Cream? Because it's no joke that Pralines 'n' Cream also has mystical healing properties."

"Agreed," I say. "But remember, we're going to resist either-or thinking."

"So what you're saying is iom2, Dreampad, and... Pralines 'n' Cream?"

"Yeah. I'm going to get my coat and we can head down to the corner store. Let's embrace CBT, ACT, *and* ICT. Ice cream therapy."

"Stan," Si says, wheeling to the front door. "I think you're really onto something here."

# 6

# A Dog With Choices

OCTOBER 17, DAY 87.

A shooting pain down the back of his right leg wakes Simon, and then me, from deep sleep.

"I'm dying here," Simon says.

I can't see the digital clock on his bedside table, but the quivering wild track of predawn birdsong outside our sliding door suggests it's the worst time to be woken abruptly: too early to rise but too late to go back to sleep. "I mean, I guess we all are," he amends. "I'm just taking a particularly harrowing route." He pops a hydromorphone, apologizes for waking me, and immediately falls back into restless slumber.

I can't go back to sleep. The tile floor of the kitchen is icy, so I pull on my slipper socks in the darkness before stumbling toward the light switch, then the kettle. It's 4:18. I make a cup of strong black tea and settle on the front porch to watch the sun rise. A tinsel spray of stars shimmers up above, and my nose and cheeks are scalded by the cold night air. Chico, only half-awake, settles down beside my wicker chair with a comically exaggerated sigh.

"I know, buddy," I say. "It's pretty early."

It's good that Simon could fall back asleep. Today is meant to be restful for him, a recovery day after the exertion of a long rehearsal with his band Farm Team last night.

*Meant to be* is the key phrase, though, as relaxing days don't really exist for him. What he needs most is a vacation from the pain—a pain-free night, or day, or afternoon, or even hour—but so far we haven't been able to make that happen. Not being able to get that simple restorative break continues to be one of the most difficult issues he faces.

It's Wednesday, so we have a TACKLING PAIN breakfast date planned for later this morning. Last week, in accordance with step two (get help!), we booked an appointment with Simon's rehab doctor, Rhonda Wilms, but her earliest available date is a month away, so we're skipping ahead to step three (confront pain). The plan so far is to carve out time for difficult conversations or, as Les Aria phrased it, *welcome the unwelcome.*

I'm anxious about what might come up.

I want to revisit a conversation that occurred in the summer, a few days before the tenth anniversary of Si's accident. It was a rare type of interaction for us: one that became heated quickly, was abruptly and unsatisfactorily ended, and had remained unresolved.

It started one afternoon when, rummaging in the messy odds-and-ends cupboard, I discovered a vial of pills tucked behind the coffee grinder. Simon was at the kitchen island, slicing crumbly old cheddar for a sandwich.

"What is this?" I asked. Pill jars generally belong to Simon, but this one was on a shelf too high for him to reach. "Oh, it's for me," I said, reading the label. The jar was full of oxycodone. "The surgeon prescribed it after the embolization." A few years before, I'd had a minimally invasive procedure to treat a uterine fibroid. It hadn't been pleasant, but neither had it been extremely painful, and I hadn't needed the pills.

The opioid crisis in British Columbia had been dominating news headlines, and after reading the many accounts of people becoming hooked on oxy after routine injuries or surgical procedures, the untouched bottle of thirty pills in my hand seemed like dangerous overkill.

"The pills are only five milligrams each," I said. "But still. It's excessive, no?"

"I don't know," Simon said, smearing Dijon across a slice of bread. "I'll take a few of those."

"What?" I said, flabbergasted. He already had a prescription for the opioid hydromorphone and took, on average, sixteen milligrams in a twenty-four-hour period. "Are you kidding? You would take unprescribed oxy? On top of your hydromorphone?"

"If it helped? Sure. In a heartbeat. To be honest, there's pretty much nothing I wouldn't do, if it took away some of this pain."

I was instantly furious. "I'm taking these into the pharmacy to dispose of," I said. "We both know that taking oxy for long-term chronic pain is more likely to make the situation worse."

Simon raised his eyebrows and tilted his head. *Do we?* But he held back from saying anything out loud.

"Listen," I said. "When we got married, I signed up for a lot of things. Better or worse. But. You choosing to take unprescribed oxy? I did not sign up for that." I glared at him. "I will not sign up for that."

"Okay, okay. I hear you," he said. "No oxy." Both of us retreated to our separate corners of the house, never to return to the subject.

Now, on this October morning as I sit on the porch sipping my tea, I wonder at the fairness of my reaction. Would an increase in Simon's opioid intake be the deal-breaker I made it out to be? No, not likely. Still, it terrifies me. Is this really his next best move?

I don't know. And I *hate* not knowing.

It's a state that certainly qualifies as being unwelcome. And, as Les Aria predicted, attempting to welcome the unwelcome only leads to other complicated emotions. Like fear. And fury.

Why am I so scared and angry? These emotions, like pain, always have a context too. When it comes to pills and booze and nicotine, I carry historical baggage. Both my parents struggled with various addictions, depression, and anxiety. Perhaps my emotional state owes more to the terrified outrage of a child watching the people she loves and depends upon make harmful choices. Simon has only ever used hydromorphone responsibly, a direct and never excessive response to very real pain. What's more harmful to him right now: opioids or the pain? It's a rhetorical question that I answer even before finishing the thought. It's the pain, absolutely.

A few weeks ago, Simon's mother, long distance from Quebec, asked if I thought Simon was suicidal. "No," I said, and I meant it. Simon has the deepest well of curiosity, wit, and playful exuberance of anyone I've ever known, and despite the extremity of his condition, that well, though diminished, was far from dry. "But," I added, knowing his mother would want the full truth, "the pain is so bad, I think he does, every day, question whether his is a life worth living." I didn't mention that recently the desperation in his offhand comments had begun to pile up.

*When the pain is this bad it makes me wonder if I should have survived my injuries.*

*I can't keep doing this.*

*I'm dying here.*

Dewy mist billows off the cedar boughs, the air iridescent with morning light. Beside me, Chico raises his head to watch a squirrel scurry across the length of our front fence and then looks back at me. *Did you see that?*

"I sure did, buddy," I say, scratching the top of his head. "And look at you, no barking. Good boy. You're a dog with choices." He thumps his tail in response to the familiar phrase: *You're a dog with choices.* It's something Simon says to him all the time, in a tone of highest compliment.

I want Simon to have choices too. Heavy doses of any opioid reduce choices. It will increase his dependency, which in turn will increase his sense of disability. I don't want those things for him, or for me. But, then again, maybe what I want is inconsequential. Maybe my expectation for his healing is an unfair burden. Maybe the only compassionate answer to his pain is drugs, and a lot of them. Maybe he's fought long and hard enough. Maybe now it's time he gets to rest.

This is not an idea that I'm comfortable contemplating. It feels like... giving up. Then there's the fact that the hydromorphone has never worked all that well at reducing his pain. At best, the pills give Simon a short-term sense of control. This is not insignificant but, over time, even this brief, chemically induced sense of agency appears to be waning. Over the past year, the pills had become less effective and his prescriptions have been running out faster each month.

This is not an uncommon situation for people using prescription opioids, and a growing body of research is delving deeper into why that might be so. New research puts forth the intriguing hypothesis that not only do opioids prolong chronic pain, they might also be a key factor in how pain becomes chronic in the first place. Studies conducted both at the Adelaide Medical School by Mark Hutchinson and at the University of Texas by Peter Grace are investigating the premise that when taken over long periods of time, opioids have at least two simultaneous and opposing actions in the body: they decrease pain via opioid receptors, but they also *increase* pain through pro-inflammatory pathways. In an acute situation, the drug's most powerful action is decreasing pain, and it is therefore highly effective in the short term. But over time that action tends to lose its efficacy. Meanwhile, the continuing activation of pro-inflammatory pathways means that the nervous and immune systems potentially become *more* sensitized to pain. It's one possible explanation of why pain can worsen even with higher and higher doses of synthetic morphine. The research continues, but the initial findings feel, at least partially, true to Simon's experience.

Were opioids, I wonder, making his pain worse?

And would Simon be open to considering that possibility?

IT'S 8:30 WHEN Simon finally rolls into the kitchen. I have a clear advantage as we sit down to our TACKLING PAIN session: I've been up for hours planning what to say while Simon, his hair mussed in sleepy tufts, is only just waking up.

"Okay, ground rules," I say. "We'll take turns sharing our most unwelcome thoughts or feelings. And that's it. No response necessary. No solutions required. The other person will listen for now. Take some time to think about it. Okay?"

"Okay."

"Do you want to start?"

"Ah, sure," Si says, yawning. "I guess the thought I'm always trying to keep at bay is how I'm letting everybody down: you, Eli, Chico, my musical pals, my family. Myself, most of all. The person I am in pain is not the person I want to be."

I bite back the urge to immediately comfort him, tell him, no, no one feels as if he's letting them down. I nod instead.

"And how about you? What's your most unwelcome thought?"

"It's complicated," I say.

"I figured." Simon smiles.

"Well, first I want to apologize for that day in the summer when I found the bottle of oxy and then freaked out."

"Okay. And...? Spill it, Stanley."

I run through the morning's most vexatious thoughts: Simon's growing desperation; my baggage concerning substance use, or misuse; the questionable efficacy and potentially hazardous long-term effects of opioids. "I don't know if it's fair or not, but I want you to keep fighting. And more opioids feel to me like you're throwing in the towel," I say. "Ultimately I want you to still be a dog with choices."

Simon grins at the reference, then sighs, admitting he too feels as if he's arrived at a crossroads with his medications. "I need to ask the doctor to up my prescription dose, but... I keep putting it off."

"Well, we don't need to come to any decision right away. Let's sit with all this for a bit. Let it soak in."

"What did you say Les Aria's phrase was? *Opening up to what's showed up*?"

"Yeah." I lean over and give him a kiss. "And that's more than enough for now."

# 7

# Grooves and Ruts

OCTOBER 24, DAY 94.

When Simon and I moved in together at the dawn of our twenties, I—a lifelong insomniac—found his ability to sleep soundly astonishing. He claimed a safe and easy passage to a land I was routinely barred from entering. He could drink a cup of coffee at ten at night and still conk out by eleven, no problem. If we had an argument between ten and eleven, he would still fall asleep. I might lie awake for hours, ruminating on his exasperation, my aggravation, trying to parse out the rightness and wrongness of it all while beside me his snores would rumble along in a bumpy purr, as if I shared a bed with some oversized adenoidal jungle cat. It was maddening.

But over the past ten years our nights have been so riddled with Simon's pain cries that I have learned the art of rolling over, huddling under the sheet, and ignoring him. I am ashamed to admit that this strategy is effective approximately 70 percent of the time. An inverse ratio is at play: the more Simon experiences the nervous system sensitization of chronic pain, the more thick-skinned and insensitive I become. Now it's me who rattles the darkness with my snores while Simon navigates the long, fretful hours of the night. Adding insult to injury, apparently I am no sweetly adenoidal jungle cat.

"More like a rutting rhino," Simon asserts. "Your snores terrify me."

But tonight, around two in the morning, a querulous treble in Simon's voice draws me out of dreamland. He has pushed himself into a seated posture and is leaning over his legs: his standard method of trying to stretch out the back spasms.

"Are you okay?"

"I'm exhausted," he says.

"Oh, Beau." Under the covers, I grab his hand and he squeezes my fingers. "I'm so sorry. I wish I could do something." A car passes on our quiet street, the headlights gliding across the blinds to the corner of the room. Beside us, on the floor, in his doggie bed, Chico snuffles and mewls, then emits a series of escalating yips.

"Easy, buddy," Simon says, lying back down. "It's only a dream."

I roll over, thinking again that, no matter how much I research, I will never fully understand what Simon's experiencing. The most current and commonly used definition of pain—"an unpleasant sensory and emotional experience associated with actual or potential tissue damage"—was crafted by the International Association for the Study of Pain. In the past, this precise, coherent description has calmed me. But it's also infuriating. *Unpleasant?* Such a tidy, neutered word.

Now I wonder, is the way the pain wakes Simon from a deep sleep, screaming, what they mean by *unpleasant?* You could say that exhaustion, despair, an ever-diminishing sense of future possibilities, and an ever-increasing sense of hopelessness are *unpleasant*, but right now in the blank space of the deep night, it's understatement to the point of mockery.

Things look better in the morning. "It's time for our weekly TACKLING PAIN meeting," I say in my UFC announcer voice.

"Yeah, well, today it's the pain that's tackling me," Si says as we sit down at the table and review the past few weeks.

Journaling, check. Simon continues to journal with his morning coffee and finds it helpful. "It's a good way to check out your internal weather on any given day," he says. "Stormy? Calm? Cloudy with a chance of meatballs?"

Curable app, check. He's committed at least five, and up to thirty, minutes a day exploring the meditation prompts. "I hate to admit it and don't you dare say *I told you so*, but focusing on your breath really does help, in the moment, to rob the pain of its looming power." He grins. "Although it must be said that Clara's voice turns distinctly sultry on the meditations. She sounds less like a friendly science nerd and more like someone on the other end of a late-night-pay-by-the-minute phone line. It's distracting."

Dreampad and iom2, check. They arrived in the mail yesterday and we're planning on spending time this afternoon getting acquainted with both products.

"Do you think we need both the iom2 *and* Curable?" I ask.

"Likely not," Si says. "It's so easy to throw money at these things and feel somehow like you're doing something, you're *investing* in being pain-free, but I don't think it's necessary. Let's cancel Curable for now. We can always pick it up again later."

And Simon has even come to at least a partial decision regarding his hydromorphone prescription: he's not going to request a higher dose. Instead, he's going to focus on building these other contingencies—breath work, meditations, journaling—and see how things go for at least the next six months. "Deal?" he says.

"Deal," I say. "Step four in our action plan was switching the focus away from the pain and on to more positive things that promote your overall health. In the ACT terminology, that would be making a commitment to engage in activities—despite the presence of pain—based on what you value the most. So. What do you value the most?"

"A clubhouse sandwich with fries. Robert Fripp's guitar solo on 'Baby's on Fire.' Stanley Cup playoff time. Beer in stubby bottles."

"That's a start."

He grins. "Okay, seriously. You, Eli. Me being a present father, husband, and musician. That's what I value," he says. "As far as specific actions, I'd like to figure out a manageable way to record the album before this year is out. I've talked to the guys. Everyone is free three weeks from now."

"It's not the graduated exposure therapy recommended by ACT, but I don't see why we can't make committing to the recording process a key intervention in TACKLING PAIN."

"Booking studio time isn't a good idea, though. It's expensive, and there's a good chance my body won't be able to handle that kind of tough schedule."

"Well, if you can't get to the studio, maybe we can bring a studio to you."

"Okay," Simon nods. "Let's do it."

MIDDAY, THREE WEEKS LATER, a Honda, its interior packed all the way to the ceiling, pulls up to the porch, and I head outside to help unload, Simon rolling behind. "Hey, brothers," Si says, beaming as the car doors open to reveal two of his all-time favorite musical collaborators: Jay Johnson and Paul Rigby. They're very different people—Jay, the drummer, is a calming, measured presence, whereas Paul, the multi-instrumentalist, projects a hummingbird energy—but they share a fluid musical intelligence. Both are fierce and creative risk takers who, amazingly, lack the overblown ego that so often accompanies that type of roving intelligence.

In addition to a drum kit, Jay's car is crammed with various guitars—an electric, an acoustic, a pedal steel—and a mandolin. And there's more: spilling from the open trunk like the unending treasures from Mary Poppins's magic bag is recording equipment, several lighting trees, long pieces of wooden doweling, and a big pink rolled-up carpet Jay bought off Craigslist.

"Hey, Jay, you checked to make sure there wasn't a body in here, right?" Paul asks, as he and I maneuver the shockingly heavy rug through the front door.

"No bodies," Jay says. "But there's a few stains better left unexplained."

We plop the rug in the living room, Simon wheeling behind.

"Hey, man." As Paul leans down and wraps his arms around Simon in a bear hug, he knocks his black trucker's cap askew, adjusting it as he stands straight. Paul always wears a hat. It's part of his musician's uniform, and is one of many reasons, big and small, that Simon and I adore him.

"I'm so glad you're here," Simon says.

"Me too. Especially as I can see you guys have already set up craft services." Paul's gaze drifts over to the long arm of our kitchen counter, which, over the next few days, I will replenish with an ongoing rotation of finger food.

"We'll pull the good stuff out later," Si says. "Right now it's just coffee and a cheese plate."

"Yum," Paul says, reaching for a mug. "It's the perfect bad breath buffet."

Jay walks by with one of the lighting trees. "That's the last of it," he says. The four of us survey the towering pile of amps, instruments, wooden doweling, and rolled-up carpet. A silky rainbow forms a secondary mound composed entirely of sleeping bags of various sizes and vintage. A faint whiff of mildew emanates from the pile.

"The Bedouin Caravan has arrived," Simon says. "And all the camels' baggage has been unloaded in our living room. What next?"

"Don't worry," Jay says. "I've got a plan."

It's precisely because of his clear vision that Jay is acting as the producer for the project. When Si called a few weeks ago to brainstorm possible solutions to his recording dilemma, Jay was immediately on board, and together he and Simon have concocted a flexible plan B.

What we need to do now is soundproof, both so outside noise doesn't get in and so inside noise is predictable and not bouncing off glass surfaces, say, or reverberating in open spaces. Jay moves decisively: first, the pink rug is unrolled. It's hideous but thankfully neither too stained nor too smelly. I add every single one of our area rugs, so that the entire living room floor is covered. Lighting trees are placed around the room, and Jay attaches the wooden doweling so that each tree is connected by a kind of makeshift curtain rod upon which we hang all our collected sleeping bags, old duvets, and raggedy blankets.

"It's the best blanket fort ever," Simon says.

We're still admiring our handiwork when Boyd Norman, the bass player, arrives. He navigates the porch steps carrying his stand-up bass, and I run to open the front door.

"Hello, Kara," he says, his starburst of a smile warming my face. It's impossible not to smile, not to pay attention, when Boyd greets you. His sentences often end in a low baritone rumble, hinting at the possibility that—no matter how prosaic the topic—he has a secret intrigue to pass on, or a hilarious joke to tell, a skill he no doubt cultivated in his many years acting on stage and radio. Boyd (like Jay and Paul) is a versatile, adaptable, spontaneous player. They're all musicians who have pulled off the rare and amazing trick of growing up without losing their childlike capacity for innovation and play.

It's wonderful to have the house suddenly filled with so much music and laughter. Over the course of the next five days, I will bear witness to a musical masterclass on the anti-perfectionist's art of improvisational magic. As much as Simon and I are committed to our TACKLING PAIN project, this musical interlude is a welcome distraction. Of course, it might also end up being a setback. Simon will undoubtedly push the limits of his physical and mental stamina over the next few days, and this increased exertion will certainly trigger escalating pain.

"I know I'll have to pay the piper eventually," Simon had said minutes before everyone arrived. "But for now I'm going to try to have fun. Hopefully I can outrun the pain long enough to capture bed tracks." It's a good bet. Despite the cost this venture will surely extract, music making is still Simon's best strategy for, well, everything.

IT WAS DURING SIMON'S REHAB, when he was healing from his brain and spinal cord injuries, that we became acquainted with the concept of neuroplasticity, the idea that our brains are constantly responding to changes in our body and in our environment. Thoughts, actions, and memories shape the very structure of the brain, as do illness, injury, stress, addictions, chronic pain, and traumatic events. Since that time, the word *neuroplasticity* has been important to us. Inside its six sturdy, evidence-based syllables, we have stuffed all our unspoken hope, fervent and fragile and tear-stained.

During rehab, hope was critical but complicated. Yes, it helped to get us both out of bed in the morning. But Simon was so vulnerable, and the implied expectation at the heart of *hope* often felt like a kind of microaggression, a suggestion that he was not whole, or complete, or enough. *Hope* was too costly a commodity. Instead we chose to fight for the more reasonable and neutral-sounding *neuroplasticity*, thus keeping our reckless hopes, if not in check, then at least safely hidden away. Neuroplasticity was our salvation. And the way to promote neuroplasticity, for Simon, was through music.

The dominant biomedical thinking of the last four hundred years has endorsed the theory that after a certain age the brain is a fixed entity, hardwired in its functions and extremely limited in its capacity to heal certain injuries. But neuroplasticity, a concept that has gained significant traction over the last fifty years, introduced the idea that our brains are engaged in a lifelong process of reaction, revision, interpretation, prediction, and adaptation. This rethinking introduces radical new implications for ideas about human healing, but the notion of neuroplasticity is not really new. At its core, it means learning. Organic, cell-deep, full-body, multidimensional meta-learning.

Neuroplasticity demonstrates that through our thoughts, actions, and experiences, we all have the capacity not only to learn throughout our lives but also to better learn *how* to learn. Your mother's admonishment that *practice makes perfect* is not so far off the Canadian psychologist Donald Hebb's explanation of one of the fundamental principles of neuroplasticity—*neurons that fire together, wire together*—which means the more your brain engages in certain kinds of thoughts, actions, or reactions, the faster, stronger, and more automatic those neural pathways become. This is true of learning specific skills, like driving a car or playing an instrument. But it's equally true for specific states, like high anxiety or vigorous enthusiasm or persistent pessimism. Our nervous system is predisposed toward efficiency because, throughout our evolutionary history, the ability to make fast decisions has been advantageous for survival. But when efficiency becomes rote repetition, our ability to discern whether these thoughts and actions are serving us is diminished. Repeated enough times, any thought, any gesture, will become normalized, a kind of default setting, even if that setting is counterproductive to our overall state of health.

Imagine the brain as a brilliant cartographer who creates a map for everything: language, movement, thoughts, feelings. Pain. When a certain map-path is traveled frequently within the brain, it becomes more and more accessible and automatic. "It's like my pain pathway used to be a dusty, barely traveled dirt trail," Si says. "Since my accident it's become a multilane mega-highway."

When Simon returned home from rehab, he had already defied everyone's expectations for his recovery, but further healing was necessary. There were occasional glitches in his memory, logic, and sequential thinking. His focus, initiative, organization, and planning skills were often a little scrambled. We didn't know whether these issues would remain, fade over time, or get worse. We suspected that rebuilding his musical skills would give him the best chance to retune his brain. Our hunch proved correct: the more he worked on the core skills of his craft, the more those post-accident cognitive glitches faded away.

Researchers today have demonstrated that intense musical training promotes neuroplasticity and strengthens sensory, cognitive, and motor functions in both the developing brain of a child and the aging brain of an adult. This is certainly true for Simon. Music allows him to continue to heal in ways both concrete and abstract. But pain is the shadow side of Simon's healing, because it too is, in part, the result of neuroplasticity. The difficult thing to understand, and accept, about the central sensitization of pain is that it's no longer an easily locatable problem. This type of pain belongs to the nervous system, and the nervous system is awesomely complex: an ongoing biological process that creates our moment-by-moment experience of being alive. As such, there is nothing to fix per se. But it can change. In fact, it insists on change. Simon is a great example of how these changeable, adaptable aspects of the human body can be both beneficial and detrimental.

"*Grooves and Ruts*," Si said a few months ago. "That's what I'm going to call the new album." As soon as he said it, it was *right*, unimaginable to have any other way. The phrase is from the final stanza of his song "Sweet Melinda":

*I'm a long way from good,*
*Man, I'm many miles from fine,*
*My records have both*
*Grooves and ruts*
*If we leave before the moon*
*We can reach the coast by noon*
*Sweet Melinda, if we only had the guts*
*Ah, Sweet Melinda, if we only had the guts.*

The inspiration for the song came when Simon was listening to Dylan's "Just Like Tom Thumb's Blues." One of the song's characters is Sweet Melinda, whom the peasants call the goddess of gloom—an unfortunate role, Simon thought, to be consigned to for the rest of eternity. His song imagines a new role for Sweet Melinda as an emblem of hope, a hands-on muse who helps the singer navigate the perils of nostalgia, regret, fear, and despair.

But it's the line *My records have both grooves and ruts* that resonates, at least for me, in a very specific way. Music is Simon's neuroplastic groove. Throughout his life, his love of music has provided shape and meaning and direction. Music is the thing he fights for, the thing that carries him through the brutally difficult days. But pain? Pain is his neuroplastic rut. Stuck inside its unyielding loop, Simon faces the loss of everything he has worked so hard to regain since his accident.

THE SOUND ENGINEER, Sasha, arrives, and as our dining room table is transformed into his recording console, Simon explains the thinking behind the most radical production decision he and Jay have made for this project: to capture the bed tracks on an analog four-track machine rather than digitally.

"I like the idea of the warmer sound," Simon says. "But more than that, it's about the process. The theme of this recording is making art with restrictions."

Capture on a four-track imposes significant restrictions. It's a type of analog technology that was cutting edge in the 1960s, when the Beatles were recording. As the name implies, there are only four available tracks: one will be used to record Boyd and Jay, bass and drums, together; another to record Paul; and the last two for Simon's vocals and guitar. It will require the band to play together, as they do when performing for an audience. And that is, in fact, what the recording will be: a chronicle of a live five-day performance in our living room. In contrast, the digital technology that revolutionized the recording industry in the 1990s offers the possibility of endless numbers of tracks. This provides vast creative opportunities, but it can often sound—at least to Simon's ears—too clinical. Too perfect.

"The ultimate criteria for the final takes we choose will be the spirit of the performance," Simon says to Sasha. "Not how pristine it is. I always loved that about bands like the Stones. Their best work—it's all about the performance. The occasional off note or weird hiccup? It makes the song more interesting."

Sasha nods but refrains from saying anything. He's not entirely convinced.

I've had my doubts too. A digital capture would provide a more reliable result. But what I love about Simon's decision is that he has taken the heartbreaking reality of not being able to record in the fully equipped studio of his choice and transformed it into a statement of creative intent. And articulating the value of creating within an anti-perfectionist framework has given Simon an impressive surge of energizing motivation. I only hope it's enough to see him through the next five days.

HE ALMOST MAKES IT. The days are long, but time rolls by quickly in a coffee-infused blur of musical exploration. Jay, Boyd, and Simon have been playing the songs as a trio now for a few months, but the addition of a gifted soloist like Paul changes the dynamic, opening new possibilities. They experiment with altering rhythm and tempo, playing with the overall feel of the songs. The four musicians share an intimate connection, finding those moments of improvisational flux, all together, a kind of communal alchemy.

As anticipated, Simon takes increasingly higher doses of hydromorphone to get through the days. "The devil's catching up to me," he says on the evening of day two, as I crawl into bed with him.

"That sounds like the start of an old blues song," I say.

"Look." He holds up his nearly empty pill jar and gives it a dismal shake. "I might have to call for an extra-early refill."

It's mid-afternoon on day four, after the third take of the high-octane song "Mr. Hopeful," when the pain overtakes Simon.

"I'm sorry, guys," he says. "I've got to lie down. I'm done for the day. This is exactly why I knew booking a pro studio was a bad idea."

He rallies for the final day, but his voice is shot and his energy is threadbare. Somehow, still, the band manages to track the final three songs.

"That's it, guys!" Simon says when they finish the umpteenth take of "Thin Air," a song that has proven frustratingly elusive. "Let's call it. We'll take a break for a few weeks, have a listening party, and then schedule in our overdubs. Yeah?"

As some of the equipment is packed away, I chop up enough lettuce to make an oversized bowl of Caesar salad and warm up a decadent tray of vegetarian lasagna donated to the recording cause by our generous neighbor Margy. A bottle of red wine is opened and a few nonalcoholic beers passed around. For a moment, the house, so full of instruments and voices, is quiet, and then Simon raises his glass to toast the band.

It's early evening when Boyd and Sasha leave for their respective homes nearby, while Jay and Paul retire to their guest rooms upstairs.

"Adult music-making camp is over," Simon says as we get ready for bed. His tone is wistful.

"You did it, Beau. Congratulations. Do you think you got everything you need for bed tracks?"

"Well, we got what we got," Simon says. "I'll think about the rest later."

In the morning, we dismantle our deluxe blanket fort, and everyone leaves.

# 8

# The Expectation Effect

NOVEMBER 13, DAY 114.

"Did you catch the game Sunday night?"

This is my cue to retreat from the conference call with Si's rehab doctor, Rhonda Wilms. The two of them—both rabid Canucks fans—commiserate on the early season performance of Vancouver's hockey team while I transfer the newly washed sheets into the dryer.

"Not bad for a pre-season skirmish," Dr. Wilms says.

"Yep. The guys looked good."

"No more Sedins," Dr. Wilms adds. "That'll make space for young blood."

"Finally," Simon says.

For over five years, Simon has checked in with Dr. Wilms every few months. So, step two (get help!) logically begins with her. Unlike many of Simon's routine medical check-ins, these appointments are something he always looks forward to. And Dr. Wilms's reciprocated pleasure in their conversation is clearly genuine. Despite her jam-packed schedule, she always makes time to connect with Simon as a whole person.

There's a recurring theme in the first-person accounts of chronic pain sufferers who have lived with a debilitating condition that has gone undiagnosed or unsuccessfully treated for months, or years. It's the significance of the moment when a medical professional stops viewing their condition as inherently suspicious and instead says: "I hear you. I believe you. I might not have any easy answers, but I believe your pain is real." And it's often this moment that marks the beginning of the movement toward healing. I suspect that this has been the case for many of Dr. Wilms's patients.

Dr. Wilms has been our most intimate ally in tackling Simon's pain, listening when we say, as we did at the outset of this conversation, that over the past year the situation has been so extreme we've both been tottering on the brink of despair. She immediately organizes a consultation with an infectious disease specialist to address the urinary tract infections, as well as one with a neuroradiologist who specializes in a nerve ablation procedure on the spinal cord.

"I'll warn you, it doesn't always work, and there are associated risks," Dr. Wilms says when I rejoin the call for its final moments. "But it sounds like we've reached a place where it's at least worth a consult."

"Agreed." Simon glances over at me, speculative hope sparking in his eyes.

"Dr. Heran's office will contact you," Dr. Wilms says. "Okay, I should let you get back to your day. What was it you said you were cooking?"

"Slow-cooked cowboy beans," Simon says. "According to the recipe, it feeds a lawyer for a day, a musician for a week, and a poet for a month."

On the other end of the line, Dr. Wilms's laughter is buoyant, unforced. It's a good note on which to end the call. We decide on a check-up in six weeks' time and say our goodbyes.

IN LATE NOVEMBER, we meet with Val Montessori, the infectious disease specialist at St. Paul's Hospital who has previously helped Simon through two potentially life-threatening MRSA infections. We're both relieved *and* happy to see her. Dr. Montessori—like Dr. Wilms—is articulate, witty, and compassionate, an example of working human intelligence at its very best. So a visit is always a pleasure—even if the circumstances suck.

"I know you two are doing everything in your power to address the recurring infections," she says, "so whatever we do here now is going to be a best-guess kind of a thing."

"It's darts at a dartboard time?" Simon says.

"Exactly."

We all agree that our first dart—a plan to put Simon on a continuous script of alternating antibiotics—is not ideal. But as Dr. Montessori points out, we've practically reached this point already over the preceding eighteen months, with the ever-decreasing window between the end of one antibiotic script and the start of a new one marked by fevers, exhaustion, and spiking pain. "We could at least eliminate the periods of infection," she says. "It might give your body a chance to recuperate."

And it does. A whole infection-free month passes, the first in almost two years. Simon's pain levels don't fade but, small mercies, he is spared the escalation that routinely occurs with a new infection. Then, in December, we travel by ferry to Vancouver for an appointment with the neuroradiologist, Dr. Heran, to discuss the proposed nerve ablation procedure.

The procedure, Dr. Heran explains, involves burning away the dorsal root ganglion at the top of Simon's lumbar spine. The dorsal root ganglion is a little bulge in the peripheral nerve at the point where it enters the spinal cord, an important hub of connection between the peripheral nerves and central nervous system. Generally, doctors fight to preserve this critical area at all cost, but because Simon is paralyzed, preserving nerve function is not the top priority.

The rationale behind the procedure is that his pain may be caused by a cluster of rogue neurons that are misfiring, blasting out danger signals despite the absence of an acute injury. All this wild misfiring provokes the intense hypersensitization of Simon's nervous system, so that over time it takes less and less stimulus to generate more and more pain.

"It's not a procedure that is done often, and the outcomes for pain relief are variable. For example, we don't know if the procedure will need to be repeated in three months, or eighteen," Dr. Heran explains. "But if it works, Simon would leave the procedural suite with no pain."

Simon and I steal a quick glance at each other. No pain? Was it even possible?

Dr. Heran's smile is warm. "I have so much respect for how you've been managing your pain, Simon. And I think we can do something to help." He hands me his card with a phone number and an email address. "Feel free to contact me if you have any further questions."

Dr. Heran's words and his kind demeanor add an effervescent sparkle to the sudden hope that surges through us both: a giddy, vibrant, loose-limbed feeling.

"What if it works? Can you imagine?" I say to Simon on the four-hour trip back home.

"No. And don't even say it out loud," Simon says. "I don't want to jinx it. After months of talking in circles about pain—"

"Hey!" I say.

"It's been good," Si adds quickly. "Don't get me wrong. But it's also hard. We put all this energy into confronting the pain, but even with our action plan it's all so abstract. I'm shadowboxing. Punching at the air. It's great to have a concrete plan. Something to *do.*"

"Yeah," I say, "but..." I'm unsure of what to say next. I don't want to be the person always dashing Simon's hopes. "Doesn't it seem almost too good to be true?"

"Listen, Stan," Si says. "Even if it's the slimmest chance of a magical medical solution, there's no discussion. I have to take it."

JANUARY 1, DAY 163.

On the first day of the new year, three months before the now-scheduled nerve ablation procedure, we sit down over blueberry pancakes to review the progress of our TACKLING PAIN project.

Things have been going well. Both the iom2 and the Dreampad have proved to be helpful. Simon particularly likes the Dreampad because it doesn't require much effort from him. He lies in bed, the pillow humming its algorithmically designed, ease-inducing sounds. There are many audio options, but, with some embarrassment, he's chosen the sound of waves: exactly the kind of soothing New Agey soundscape that he mocked ferociously throughout his twenties.

"I get a big pain spike transitioning from the wheelchair into bed," he tells me, "so it's not like it's immediately taking away the pain. But... it's inexplicable. The sound of the waves is warm. When I first lie down, I always feel angular and harsh. Jangly. But by the end of the half hour I'm... calmer. All my edges are a little softer."

The iom2 has been a success as well, although it requires a little more effort. Similar to an iPod, the iom2 is a simple biofeedback device. It has a sensor (which can be attached to an earlobe or fingertip) that measures something called heart rate variability, or HRV—the lapses of time *between* the beats of the heart. This physiological measurement is one of the best ways of gauging the overall resilience of the nervous system, indicating how easily a person can move back and forth between the sympathetic mode of fight-or-flight and the parasympathetic rest-and-digest. Generally, the HRV measurement plummets in someone with a condition like chronic pain, indicating an overstressed system that lacks adaptability.

The iom2 connects to an online app that provides a series of mindfulness prompts, or "Zen journeys." Simon prefers these prompts to Curable's because there are several different speaking voices to choose from and the audio is accompanied by vivid images of various landscapes. To advance, or level up, in your Zen journey, you need to increase your HRV, which is described within the app as your "resonance score." Simon was fascinated to discover that when he intentionally focuses on his breath, he can affect his HRV. He's been not-so-subtly bragging about it for the past month.

"So, basically," I said one day as he crowed over a dramatic spike in his resonance, "you needed mindfulness to be measured for it to be interesting."

"Competitive mindfulness," he joked. "You might have something there."

With the help of these interventions he's been able to resist asking the doctor to up the dose of his opioid prescription. He hasn't decreased his hydromorphone use, but it hasn't increased either. And he's maintained his morning journaling, although, as the recording project has progressed, he's used that writing time to brainstorm, troubleshoot, and make album-related to-do lists.

"If a pain thought or feeling comes up," he says now, "I'll get it down. But it's good to have my mind preoccupied with something else."

"Definitely. So, one last thing..." I say, hesitating. I'm not sure how to proceed. The next topic falls directly into the "make room for difficult conversations" category, but I'm struggling with what, and how much, to say.

Simon is enthusiastic about the upcoming nerve ablation procedure. But over the Christmas holidays I started to entertain serious doubts. I worry that the nerve ablation won't work, or that if it does, the effects will only last a very short time and we'll become locked into an exhausting and ultimately unsustainable routine of surgical interventions every few months. It's exactly the type of scenario we hoped to avoid with step one of our action plan: let go of the idea of a single solution. Simon and I have come to a hard-won understanding that his pain is not located solely in specific tissues. Instead we imagine it more as an out-of-control wildfire flaring through his whole nervous system. In my most doubtful moments, I worry that burning away a small area of tissue in the dorsal root ganglion is equivalent to shooting a water pistol at a single tree and hoping to douse a thousand acres. Perhaps the nerve ablation might have been effective ten years ago, when Simon's pain was just a small spark. But now, after a decade of continuing changes to his central nervous system, is there any chance that it will work?

Simon has many animated telephone conversations with his mother, Lorna, about the potential of the upcoming procedure. His spinal cord injury was classified as complete, which means that the spinal cord is entirely severed. This was true in clinical terms—he is what physical therapists refer to as a floppy paraplegic, with 100 percent motor and sensory loss below his level of injury—but the cord was not totally severed; it was *almost* totally severed. A thin sliver, compressed and damaged, remained intact. For many years, Lorna has been convinced that severing the last bit of spinal cord would stop the pain. As far as she's concerned, this logical next medical intervention should have happened years earlier.

But phantom body pain in paraplegic patients confounds logical thought. Like Les Aria, both Patrick Wall and Ron Melzack believed this to be one of the most mysterious of all pain phenomena. In their groundbreaking book *The Challenge of Pain,* they describe the potentially dire results of the kind of mechanistic, logical thinking that Lorna is so certain is the answer to Simon's pain.

One case study tells the story of DG, who fractured vertebrae in a car accident and became paraplegic. Within a year of his accident he began to suffer from crushing, knife-like sensations in his chest, torquing cramps in his abdomen, and burning spasms in his legs and hips. Anesthetic blocks were administered on several occasions, along with various analgesic drugs. Nothing worked. Next a cordotomy was performed: a neurosurgeon excised a part of the spinal cord called the spinothalamic tract, a key pathway in processing pain. Still, the burning, cramping, knife-twisting sensations continued. Next, a rare and desperate surgery—a cordectomy—was carried out, a neurosurgeon removing a section of the spinal cord at the level of DG's original injury. In the immediate aftermath, DG experienced a reduction in the crushing pain in his chest, but his abdominal and hip pain remained unaltered. And even this partial relief was only temporary. Eight months after the operation, and despite the many stressful and risky interventions, his pain profile had returned to the pre-intervention state.

More heartbreaking still was the case study of a man who suffered a brachial plexus avulsion, meaning that the network of nerves that provide movement and feeling to his shoulder, arm, and hand were torn at the spot where they attached to his spinal cord, so that his entire arm was paralyzed. After the injury, he developed phantom pains in his unfeeling limb. To treat the pain, his arm was amputated, and when that didn't work, neurosurgeons performed a high cervical cordotomy, again excising sections of the spinothalamic tract. When the first cordotomy failed, they did a second, more extensive one. Next a series of operations were performed on his brain, first in the frontal lobes and then in his thalamus. But none of these aggressive interventions reduced the pain. Desperate and feeling he was out of viable options, this man died by suicide.

These stories haunt me. And the more I think about it, the more the upcoming procedure—scheduled in three months' time—provokes a visceral horror: we are willfully agreeing to inflict more damage on Simon's already damaged nervous system. It's a desperate decision.

But that's the thing. Despite the progress we've made, Simon *is* desperate. We both are. And it's hard to trust your internal voices when you're desperate. Visceral horror was what I experienced when Simon underwent emergency brain and spinal cord surgeries, but these same surgeries granted him the slimmest percentage of survival. And Simon's recovery defied the odds. Despite grave injuries, his body was resilient. Maybe, with Dr. Heran's help, he could defy the odds one more time. But, then again, Simon has endured so much over the past ten years. How much more can he take?

All month long this is how it's gone: questions without answers; thoughts that flip-flop between horror and hope.

Worst of all, I've actively restrained myself from discussing all of this with Simon. And that is largely due to the research I've been reading on the placebo effect.

The negative connotations of the word *placebo* have deep roots. Latin for "I shall please," it came into regular usage in the fourteenth century to refer to professional mourners, often priests or friars, who were paid to chant, sing, and mourn for the dead. The "singing of placebos" was thought—at least by Chaucer—to be an act of insincere flattery, and he named a character in *The Canterbury Tales*, a notorious sycophant, Placebo. Since then the word has connoted a sense of fakery—something that while superficially pleasing is void of substance.

Dating back to our medical forefathers, Hippocrates and Galen, it has long been acknowledged that physicians could affect healing using non-pharmacological interventions such as bread pills, sugar tablets, colored water, and ashy powders made of ground tree bark. In 1785 George Motherby's *A New Medical Dictionary* defined *placebo* as "a common place method or medicine." In 1811 *Hooper's Medical Dictionary* updated the definition, stating that a placebo was "any medicine adapted more to please than benefit the patient." Eleven years earlier, in 1800, a brief but remarkable treatise had been published, called *Of the Imagination, as a Cause and as a Cure of Disorders of the Body, Exemplified by Fictitious Tractors, and Epidemical Convulsions.* The author, John Haygarth, was a British physician who originally set out to impartially investigate the claims of an American doctor, one Elisha Perkins, and, in doing so, discovered something quite unexpected.

Dr. Perkins had invented Perkins Patent Tractors, two three-inch steel or brass rods that tapered to a blunt point at one end. Small, unobtrusive, and seemingly without any practical purpose, they resembled a miniature set of knitting needles. Perkins declared that the special properties of his metal alloys allowed him to cure inflammation, rheumatism, gout, toothaches, and headaches by placing the points of the rods directly on the aching body part. Despite being derided as quackery by the medical community, the high-priced Tractors were a hot commodity.

Haygarth designed a series of trials to test the efficacy of the real metal tractors against a variety of imitations made from a range of other substances: mahogany, iron nails covered in sealing wax, bone, an old tobacco pipe, a pair of slate pencils. It turned out that all the imposters were as effective in producing relief as the metal tractors, providing an important lesson for Dr. Haygarth, who wrote that "the wonderful and powerful influence of the passions of the mind upon the state and disorder of the body [is]... too often overlooked in the cure of diseases." He concluded that the powers of the imagination were yet imperfectly understood and constituted a valid and rich area of further medical inquiry.

Still, the routine use of placebos throughout the nineteenth century was not believed to have any real physiological impact. Rather, it was viewed as an effective strategy to placate difficult patients while the healing power of time took its natural course. The more powerfully a placebo worked, the more poorly it reflected on the moral integrity and intelligence of the patient. According to a historical overview of the medical use of placebos published in the *Journal of the Royal Society of Medicine*, those susceptible to the sham effects of a fake drug were considered "unintelligent, neurotic, or inadequate patients" (a Victorian phrase we can now roughly translate as most often referring to women).

Placebos are still important today in medical research. Any new medication is tested against a placebo and needs to be demonstrably more effective to be approved. In randomized double-blind studies, neither the researcher nor the study participant knows who is receiving the placebo and who is receiving the real medication. Irene Tracey, head of the neurosciences department at the University of Oxford, calls this testing phase the "graveyard of drug discovery" in the pain field because it's rare that a new drug outperforms the placebo.

In *Pain: The Science of Suffering,* Patrick Wall recounts a study performed at Eastman Dental Hospital in London that eerily echoes Haygarth's trial of Perkins Patent Tractors. The patients in the study had recently undergone a wisdom tooth extraction; their faces were swollen and sore, and they were reluctant to open their mouths. In the first phase, a doctor explained that ultrasound had been proven to reduce inflammation, and then proceeded to massage the patient's face with an ultrasound machine. This proved to be highly effective in reducing healing time.

For the next phase, the double-blind, the doctors massaged the patients' faces with an ultrasound machine that in some cases was turned on and in others wasn't, unbeknownst to both doctor and patient. Again, there was a marked improvement in healing but, strangely, there was no difference between the two groups.

For the final phase, the patients were requested to self-administer the ultrasound massage without the doctor's help. This time no healing benefits occurred. The results of the study were clear: the placebo effect was potent. It had reduced not only pain (a subjective measure) but also inflammation (an objective measure), the placebo's action being equivalent to a substantial dose of an anti-inflammatory steroid. But to work, the placebo effect required an impressive machine (whether it was on or off) wielded by a person invested with medical authority.

Since that time, advances in neuroimaging technology have allowed us to better understand placebos. Some of the latest research is being directed by Dr. Tracey in her labs at Oxford. She and her team conducted brain-imaging studies on healthy participants who were simultaneously subjected to painful stimuli and given a powerful intravenous pain-killing opioid. The researchers began by starting the intravenous injection without alerting the participants. Next they claimed to start the opioid injection even though participants were already on the drug. Then finally, they told the participants they were stopping the drug when in fact they weren't. "The results," Dr. Tracey reports, "were striking." Although the hidden injection had a minor analgesic effect, that effect was doubled when the participants were told the drug was going to start—even though they had already been receiving it for some time. And, perhaps most strikingly, *all* analgesic effect was canceled when the researchers pretended to stop the infusion. Even though the test participants were still receiving the same dose of the opioid, they now rated their pain the same as they had before any infusion of the drug.

The brain-imaging studies revealed that it was the participants' shifting expectations rather than the opioid infusion that shaped their experience of pain. When the expectations were positive (placebo), the nervous system worked to inhibit pain, and when the expectations were negative (nocebo) the nervous system amplified pain.

Biologically speaking, Dr. Tracey concluded, nothing special was occurring. Powerful expectations had the ability to hijack the nervous system, in both positive and negative ways. But the implications were groundbreaking: it is possible to shape people's expectations, and thereby their experience of pain. Perhaps, Dr. Tracey suggested, placebos were an overlooked tool in the fight against chronic pain. And so, she has proposed a rebranding: Forget the *placebo effect* and its centuries-long association with quacks, charlatans, and fakers. Now it's time for the *expectation effect.*

Unlike drugs, surgeries are rarely tested against a placebo, as surgical interventions are assumed to work. Dr. Tracey suggests that this is a big assumption, and work in her labs, and elsewhere, is demonstrating that the expectation effect is active even in a surgical context. In 2014, the *British Medical Journal* published a study investigating whether placebo controls should be used to evaluate the effectiveness of certain surgical procedures. The overwhelming finding was yes. The researchers concluded that the placebo effect influenced a wide range of surgeries, but its effects were most noticeable, and long lasting, when the surgery was primarily intended to address something that relied on a patient's subjective report—like, say, persistent pain.

What did that mean for Simon? How relevant are Dr. Tracey's experiments to his experience of pain? In the intravenous opioid experiment, her test subjects were healthy. Likely they were university students who had willingly signed up. Perhaps they were curious about the process or received class credit. Or maybe the promise of a strong dose of opioids was intriguing enough.

The students would also have entered the experience knowing a few things: first, that the researchers could not ethically inflict long-lasting harm, so whatever pain they were about to feel posed no meaningful threat. Also, and perhaps most important, they would have known that if they became too uncomfortable at any time, they could stop. All of these factors—the willing consent, the lack of real threat, the acute, transitory nature of the pain, the finite nature of the experiment, and the ability to call a halt to it at any time—create a bedrock of expectations that are essentially the opposite of Simon's daily experience. For Simon, pain is amorphous, quixotic, violent, unending. Despite our best efforts and those of the medical community, it is still uncontrollable and essentially unknowable. He did not sign up for it. All of these factors create a very different set of underlying expectations. How, I wonder, would they affect Simon's surgical outcomes?

The only thing clear to me is this: I have no idea.

I want to do what's best for Simon, but what is that? Given my research on the expectation effect, it's not lost on me that, though I'm skeptical of her logic, Lorna's confidence and eager enthusiasm about the upcoming surgery might contribute to a more positive outcome.

But I can't lie to Simon. I won't say I'm confident and enthusiastic when in fact I'm filled with horror and doubt. I review the facts, the most important being that Simon, even after hearing about the lack of guaranteed results, is unwavering: this is what he wants.

Do I honestly believe that the expectation effect might be the only benefit of the procedure? No. I know from my research that the dorsal root ganglion is a critically important area in the modulation of pain. I had worried that this potentially risky procedure was the equivalent of shooting a water pistol at a tree while the whole forest burned. But perhaps a more appropriate analogy might be turning off a gas stove that had been left on; the house might still be burning, but with the gas off, we would finally have a chance at controlling the fire.

The basic premise of our pain project has been that no single, surefire solution exists for treating pain. Simon and I both believe that, as is often the case in creative pursuits, sometimes two plus two comes closer to equaling five. That is, the synergy of forces might create something greater than the sum of its parts. Maybe effective treatment for Simon's pain requires all these things: surgery, the expectation effect, journaling, meditation, and... what else?

It's this *what else?* that starts to tip me into a more positive way of thinking. The ablation procedure will take place in three months. Are there other things we could do in that time to increase the chances that the fire will die down when the burner is switched off?

"DO YOU FEEL like I'm being too bossy with all the pain stuff?" I ask now as we linger over a second cup of coffee. This is something else that has been troubling me over the holidays: over the past few months, the balancing act of our marriage has become precariously out of whack. Right now, I'm the active agent constantly pushing to address the problem of pain. Simon is more passive, a role both unusual and ill-fitting for him. Within this teeter-tottery relationship equilibrium, I'm never sure if I'm pushing too hard, or not hard enough. Pain research underscores that people who take control of managing their own pain have better outcomes, and I don't want to impede Simon's sense of agency by being overbearing. But, also, I know Simon and I know right now, more than at any other time in our marriage, he needs help. He needs structure; he needs a push.

"Bossy-bossy-two-by-four?" he singsongs. It's a family take on a familiar schoolyard taunt, one we all sang when Eli was younger as a playful shorthand to politely tell someone to back off.

"Yeah, exactly. Am I being a bossy-bossy-two-by-four?"

"Yes. No." He smiles. "Remember when you said you worried that your attitude toward pain was about as helpful as telling a drowning man to learn to swim? Well, I feel like the last few months have been the equivalent of being tossed a flutterboard, and... I need that assist. Hopefully, soon, I'm swimming on my own. But for now, it really helps. Plus, you know, you're pretty cute with your bossy-pants on."

"All right. I'm glad we're on the same page, because I wanted to broach something tricky."

"Uh-oh."

"Ssshh," I say, waving my hand with bossy-bossy imperiousness. "It's this: you've put in so much work over the last few months, and I know there's no instant improvement, but... it does seem like things are incrementally better. Would you agree?"

He nods, shoveling in a last bite of syrup-soaked pancake.

"I don't want to be discouraging, but I think all those things are a baseline," I say. "You've got to maintain the breathing practice and the Dreampad and the writing. But we need to keep going. Look at more specific things we can do to help with neuroplasticity. We can think about it as a kind of preparation, to give your nervous system the best possible chance to benefit from the ablation procedure."

"It's a good idea," he says.

"Yeah? Really? You think so?"

"Yeah. I'm with you, Stanley. Let's do it."

# 9

# The King of Fake News

FEBRUARY 6, DAY 199.

When pain persists for no known reason, there are two likely scenarios. The first is rare: an underlying cause *does* exist but has yet to be discovered or understood—for example, an undiagnosed infection, autoimmune disorder, or tumor. The second, and more common, scenario is that the nervous system has been so overwhelmed (by a complex multitude of factors that range from the physiological to the psychological to the social) that it becomes hypervigilant, perceiving threat where none may exist. In this instance the relationship between tissue injury and pain falls perilously out of sync.

After a decade's immersion in the health care system, Simon and I have learned a hard truth: neither routine medical practices nor the way our culture conceptualizes pain are conducive to supporting the health of our nervous system. Pain is a great disruptor—but pain is not the only thing that disrupts our nervous system. There is a compelling argument to be made that human cultural and technological advances have outpaced our evolutionary biology. Our nervous systems are hardwired to focus on any threatening aspect of our environment, an adaptive trait that greatly increased the survival chances of your average hunter-gatherer. But now our biology is often in discord with the constant stimulation, and potential threat, of our fast-paced but sedentary, round-the-clock digitized lives: physical bodies clashing with the tech-driven world we have created. Modern life routinely overwhelms even the most robust of nervous systems.

Neuroplastic healing is tricky because the nervous system doesn't belong to a single physical structure. It has several complex parts—the brain, the brain stem, the spinal cord, and the many peripheral nerves threaded throughout the body. In this way, it is perhaps more accurate to conceive of it not as a locatable *thing* but as a *process*, an ongoing process that is responsible for creating the moment-by-moment experience of being alive.

The overall resiliency of this process has an enormous impact on how we move, think, and feel. There is truly nothing to lose and everything to gain by addressing nervous system health—for everyone, but especially the person-in-pain. Of course, the really difficult question is *how?* How do you cross-train, pump up, or tone your nervous system? Simon and I spend long hours discussing this conundrum and conclude that there will be as many answers to the question as there are people in the world. The real challenge for us all—whether we're currently in pain or not—is to stay connected and grounded in an increasingly fragmented and fractious world. It's critical to cultivate restorative spaces of safety, pleasure, and connection. Critical, too, to honor your body. Simon's nervous system is doing its very best under extraordinarily challenging circumstances. This is true of anyone experiencing pain.

THE CENTRAL TENET of the *Neuroplastic Transformation* workbook is that although neuroplastic change is responsible for transforming the symptom of acute pain into the disease of chronic pain, it is also the solution to restoring health. The workbook identifies sixteen areas in the brain that are involved in pain perception, only nine of which are under our conscious control. In a healthy state, approximately 5 percent of the nerve cells within these nine areas are dedicated to processing pain, but in a persistent state, this rises to as high as 25 percent.

This is how the brain learns pain—by claiming more and more cortical real estate. It has turned Simon's dusty pain-path into a multilane freeway. The challenge in unlearning pain is to block that traffic, reducing the busy highway back to a quiet trail. This, the handbook suggests, can be accomplished by consciously countering every single episode of pain with a non-painful stimulus. As the authors, Michael Moskowitz and Marla Golden, state:

> We can create and effect changes in our brain and our lives through repetitive thoughts of reducing the pain, soothing emotions and sensations and comforting beliefs. Vision, scent, touch, sound, movement, meditative calm, spirituality, kindness, gratitude and love all directed toward changing the brain allow us to change cells, genes, molecules, anatomy, physiology and circuits. We shift the balance away from unrelenting pain to normal brain function. We reclaim what we have lost.

Some concrete suggestions to accomplish this difficult task include "gently stroking the skin, listening to soothing music, progressive muscle relaxation, smelling a pleasing scent, breathing exercises, recalling a pleasurable experience, looking through old pictures." Simon and I have already spent an afternoon brainstorming our own additional interventions.

It's not our first time doing this. I ordered the book three years ago, and Simon and I spent a wet West Coast winter poring over its pages. But we agree that revisiting the handbook now might be a whole new experience. The main problem is that in the face of his formidable pain, the neuroplastic strategies all feel a little... feeble. Ridiculous, even.

"Apparently, believing that chronic pain is *not* inevitable is key to a neuroplastic intervention. Eliminating pain has to be the goal, not self-management," Simon says, after his second read-through. "It's like the Curable app says: You have to *want* to *believe* you can get better," Simon singsongs in an approximation of Clara's affable feminine voice. "As if ongoing pain is a failure of *wanting* and *believing*."

"Hmmm," I say.

"I feel like there's a lot behind that *hmmm*," Si says.

"Well. I'd say—and I think the workbook would agree—*experiencing* is always more important than *wanting* or *believing*."

"Interesting," Simon says, nodding. "Explain."

It's a long explanation, one that involves my own history. A childhood horseback riding accident, a congenital malformation in my spine, and long workdays sitting in front of a computer had wreaked havoc on my lower back, and I spent all of my thirties in considerable distress. For me, the solution was a committed movement practice. I studied, then trained as a teacher in, the Classical Pilates method, steadily progressing through safe, then pleasurable, then empowering movement. Before Si's accident, the debilitating soreness had been a part of my life for so long, it had begun to feel intrinsic to me. I wasn't pleased with it, but, like being nearsighted or shy or having a sweet tooth, it was, for better or worse, who I was. Low back pain had somehow morphed into a self-defining trait; I thought it was a permanent part of my personality. But now that's changed.

I had entered the Pilates studio rooted in a core belief that pain—all pain—was bad, dangerous, threatening. But now I would say this: movement—the right kind of movement—heals. Sometimes, when you're beginning to move, pain is a normal, appropriate, and expected sensation. The only way to get to the other side is through it. Dedicating myself to a movement practice wasn't a quick-fix solution—it took almost three years to fully shift out of low back pain—but it opened the way for a transformative process that continues today.*

"My first few Pilates sessions started out so slowly, with such gentle, progressive movements, that it gave me an opportunity to experience my body as not feeling broken, or in danger," I say to Simon now. "Every little sliver of feeling better, or safer, became something to build on. And that's my approach for teaching: sometimes a student will show up feeling grumpy or tired or fearful. Advising them to not feel that way wouldn't be very effective. But if I can help them *experience* safe, pleasurable, or empowering movement,

* The online Pain Resource Guide (see page 330) provides an expanded discussion on the importance of a movement practice. Various movement modalities are discussed, along with a list of helpful hints to aid in choosing the right method and teacher for *you*.

there's usually a rapid shift to a more positive state of being. So. I don't know..." I conclude vaguely. "What do you think? Is a pain-free intention helpful for you, or not?"

"In the moment, when the pain hits, it's not so much that it's helpful or harmful, it's just absurd," Simon says. "It's like you've got a shark attacking you and someone is saying, to get that shark to stop attacking you, what you have to do is believe that one day a shark will not be attacking you. You have to *want* to *believe* that one day a shark will not be attacking you. But in the moment, none of that matters. Because... a fucking shark is attacking you."

"I feel that way about some of the proposed neuroplastic interventions," I say. "That shark is biting you and I'm standing there daubing a hemorrhaging wound with a cotton swab, saying, *breathe, just breathe*. But we know these interventions take time. Three months at least. We can't do it once, feel silly, then never do it again. None of it is going to work overnight."

"Right."

"We have to stick with it."

"Right."

"And I want to be able to help. But... I worry that if I cue you to breathe, or ask you a math question, or tickle your nose, you're going to feel like I'm trivializing your pain. I don't want that."

"Well... maybe we need a pain safe word?" Si says. "In case the intervention is making things worse, not better."

"Like what?"

"How about 'No no no' or 'Stop'?"

"Both are preferable to 'fuck off,'" I say. "Which, under the circumstances, also seems reasonable."

Simon smiles over his shoulder. "I appreciate that."

He cracks open a tall bottle of Stella Artois and pours it into two glasses. It's a small pleasure that's been denied to him for many years, as beer—even the smallest amount—seemed to directly contribute to his urinary tract infections. But now that the UTIs are being successfully managed with weekly antibiotics, we're experimenting with the occasional evening libation.

"Cheers, baby," he says, and we clink glasses. "A few songs before dinner?"

We start with Gillian Welch and Dave Rawlings's "Hard Times," which Simon plays at a sprightlier pace than the original. As we sing, the music works its magical algebra: the more we pour ourselves into the song, the more it gives back. Three songs is about Simon's max before the pain starts to bark, and so after a rendition of Dylan's "One More Cup of Coffee" and Patsy Cline's "Walkin' After Midnight," I suggest we call it.

"I have one more song in me," Si says.

"Let's stop before the pain hits," I say. "Keep it in the pleasure zone." This is a major component of the *Neuroplastic Transformation* workbook: counter pain with pleasure. While Simon is often dubious about certain aspects of our project, he is uniquely committed to this strategy.

"Right, the pleasure zone," he says, with a lascivious wink. "What do you say, shall we engage in a little competitive neuroplasticity in the pleasure zone later this evening?"

THIS IS HOW SIMON AND I BEGIN: we print out two contrasting images showing a side view of a brain. The first image shows the regions of the brain used to perceive pain lit up with a white-gold light. The second image shows undisturbed brain tissue, with no pain sunspots visible.

The workbook advises looking at the pain-free graphic and thinking, "If my brain looks like this, I can feel no pain." This, the workbook tells us, "stimulates visual processing, which in turn activates problem solving, planning, conflict resolution, autobiographical memory, emotional regulation and pain relief." It seems a lot to expect from a simple picture of a brain.

This was the technique detailed in Norman Doidge's *The Brain's Way of Healing* and used by Michael Moskowitz to heal his own persistent neck pain. He countered every incursion of pain with this visualization of the brain. I wonder if it might work for Simon. We make copies of these images, gluing them into his journal and hanging them in almost every room of the house so that Simon can look at them whenever the pain strikes.

A few weeks later, when I'm sweeping, I find two of the pictures under the kitchen table.

"Throw 'em out," Simon says. "They bug me. I prefer to think of pain like an oil spill. Like BP in the Gulf of Mexico. And then I imagine big oil booms containing, then shrinking, the spill."

"Does it help?" I ask, noting but not saying out loud that Simon's visual metaphor includes shrinking and containing but not totally eradicating the pain.

"Mhhhmph," Si says. He smiles. "Maybe a bit. But not really. Not yet."

We fill a diffuser with peppermint oil—the scent of peppermint helps block substance P, a main neurotransmitter associated with pain. At night, when we switch on the diffuser, I say, *the smell of peppermint is going to block your substance P, which is going to reduce your overall pain, and you are going to have a better sleep tonight*. *Yes*, Simon answers (because I insist), *the substance P will be blocked, my pain will be less, and I will sleep better.* We say the same thing every night so that it becomes a kind of joke, but I'm also deadly serious. My earnestness makes Simon laugh. The pervasive smell of peppermint is not unpleasant.

Our brainstorm sheet has many suggestions that Simon vetoes immediately. Like idea #7: learn a complex piece of choral music and sing when the pain gets bad.

"Even if it's the middle of the night," I say, trying to be helpful.

"No," Simon says.

I purchase a roll-on aromatherapy tube of peppermint oil so that Simon can dab it on his nostrils when taking his medication. By doing this we hope to amplify the effect of his pain-relieving meds as well as set up a conditioned response so that eventually, just dabbing his nose will provide a measure of relief. Next, we compile a list of questions that I can prompt Simon with when the pain howls. We target two key areas, problem solving and autobiographical memory. Many of the latter questions focus on the late seventies, when Simon was a young child. His family lived in Jamaica for three years, and it was an era of brightly distinct memories.

*Describe your first-grade teacher*, I ask as he screams.

*What was it like to snorkel at Dragon Bay?*

*Walk me through your house in Jamaica.*

The workbook also recognizes the importance of the tenth cranial, or vagus, nerve, noting that the most all-encompassing circuit in the brain is that of sound. Some electrochemical rhythms of the brain can be reproduced in music. "One beat per second is the frequency nerve cells use to slow down and stop constantly firing," the workbook tells us. "One beat every two seconds is the rhythm used by nerves in the part of the brain known as the hippocampus to release GABA into emotional circuits to calm anxiety. One beat every three seconds is the speed at which nerve cells fire when at rest." Simon downloads the recommended recording titled "Brain Music: Default Mode Network," a series of slow, deep frequencies meant to calm an overly active brain and help reduce anxiety. We switch the iPad on as we turn off the lights. "Oh boy," Simon says when he hears the low gong of Tibetan singing bowls. "All those sounds are in F. I don't know about this." Despite his apprehension, we both fall asleep quickly.

"What do you think?" I ask in the morning.

"Meh," he says. "At least it didn't keep me up."

"Let's stick with it," I say. I'm pumped. I had the best sleep I've had in years.

SIMON READS ME an entry in his journal:

> *Ah, the Brain: King of Fake News; The Great Deceiver; Suggestive Side Street Swinger. Listen up! I am conducting a self-regulated experiment. Perhaps peppermint scent, hippie trance music, creative visual imagery, and dogmatic mantras will help to re-program you, my poor misguided brain. You are so intent on serving only one master—Pain. But my intention is to dethrone this master, revealing him to be smoke and mirrors, his illusionary power utterly reliant on these crooked cognitive embellishments. I will question my own body's "rule of law," finally proving that the Emperor Pain wears no clothes. Pain, I'm done with your bullshit. From here on in it's going to be better quality of life: pleasure,*

*pleasure, pleasure. Less medications; more music and love and light and grace.*

"It's lyrical," I say.

"But so far the coup has been unsuccessful," he says.

Still, we're figuring a few things out. We discover that the distracting questions or activities must be easy enough that Simon can turn his full attention to them even during a flare-up of pain, but not so easy that they don't pose some form of challenge. Our most inventive idea is to learn sign language. We spend a fun evening practicing how to sign the alphabet with an online tutorial and coming up with lewd-but-satisfying phrases to describe Simon's pain. *You skitchy strumpet; you bull-pizzle; you fucking pisspot.* Simon loves Ian McShane's character Al Swearengen in the series *Deadwood*. Our goal: to cuss like Swearengen in sign language. A good idea, but it fails in practice. "Stop, just stop!" Simon shouts at me, when I urge him—like some frenetic birth coach—to breathe and sign during a pain contraction.

So far, the most successful distraction is when I ask him to solve double-digit multiplication tables. No matter how bad his pain is, Simon can't *not* answer a math challenge. Although it doesn't take the pain away entirely, we're both impressed with how effective it is immediately—if briefly—in turning the volume down.

It's small, but it's something.

# 10

# Breathe—Just Breathe

MARCH 13, DAY 234.
*Three weeks before nerve ablation procedure.*

TWO PERCENT, TO BE PRECISE. Simon figures the neuroplastic strategies have eased the pain by two percent.

It's happy hour, and we're seated in a busy restaurant around the corner from our Vancouver hotel. It's a rare indulgence these days, eating out at a restaurant, and we're trying to make the most of it. Simon digs into the second half of his club sandwich while I delicately refrain from licking the remnants of a shrimp paella off my plate.

"Two percent, hey?" While neither of us was expecting instantaneous results—*it takes time*, we kept reminding each other, *like learning a new instrument*—it's disarmingly small progress to show for our weeks of round-the-clock commitment to countering the pain. In Norman Doidge's *The Brain's Way of Healing*, Michael Moskowitz suggests that when patients don't benefit from his neuroplastic techniques, it's because they've been unable to mobilize themselves mentally for the challenge.

Is that us? Unable to mobilize for the challenge? I don't think so. Simon might have fared better with a team of neuroplastic interventionists to support and guide him, instead of just me, but is that even a job? Neuroplastic interventionist? It's certainly not been on our menu of treatment options. We're coming to realize that the *neuroplastic learning* in Simon's long and difficult recovery from traumatic brain injury might have been a breeze compared with the *neuroplastic unlearning* required to heal a state of chronic pain.

"I know it seems small," Si says. "But, you know, even a small improvement is huge."

"Well done!" The waitress says, clearing our bare plates away. "Do you want dessert?"

It's tempting. It's been a difficult day. When we arrived at the hotel to check in, we were told that the wheelchair-accessible room we had booked three months ago was no longer available. Those who don't travel with a wheelchair might be surprised that this frequently happens. The hotel gives away the room to someone else who needs accessible accommodations. Since Si's accident, we've run into this issue, or a critical problem with the safety of a so-called accessible room, on at least 80 percent of our travels.

What was most irritating today was that the young clerk had, instead of admitting the error, insisted that it was in fact hotel policy: accessible rooms could not be guaranteed until check-in. His name tag identified him as Andy; he was smug, with a thin smile plastered across his round face throughout our exchange.

"So, that means if you are a person with a high-level spinal cord injury traveling from Prince George to Vancouver," I challenged him, "you won't know if you have an accessible room until you check in and are miles away from home?"

"Yes," Andy insisted, smile tightening. In my most reasonable, older-sister voice, I told him this was ludicrous.

After a quick conference, Si and I decided that to deal with the situation without losing our minds we first needed food, and so we accepted the key card for the non-accessible room conditionally, both of us using our best no-bullshit voices to let Andy know that there was no way this was official hotel policy. We'll be returning now to that non-accessible room, where Simon can manage to transfer into the bed but can't access the bathroom, and our evening will be spent trying to secure accessible accommodations for after Simon's day surgery tomorrow.

"I'm stuffed," Si says to the waitress.

"Me too," I say. "Thanks, but we'll take the check."

THE NEXT DAY, at break of dawn, we make our way to the hospital. Renovations are underway at the hotel, requiring us to park our wheelchair van in another underground lot. We decide it's faster, and easier, to walk the five-odd blocks to the hospital than to retrieve the van. I enjoy the walk. It's rare for us to be outside, together, this early in the morning. A thread of bright pink hems the lavender sky and a cool, salt-tinged sea breeze ruffles down the still empty city streets. But there is little pleasure for Simon in our jaunt. Every bump in the cracked and uneven sidewalk sets off spasms so intense he can't roll on his own. I push the chair as he groans over each rattling jolt, the breath catching in the back of his throat.

"Maybe we should have brought the van," I say, as we wind up the ramp to the front doors of the hospital.

"No," Si says. He takes over wheeling the chair, gliding through the front doors over the smooth, even floors. "This made more sense." Today Dr. Heran will perform a spinal angiogram, threading a small catheter into Simon's right femoral artery, the main artery that supplies blood to the leg. Because it's so close to the surface of the skin, it's often the site where catheters are inserted. From this insertion site, soft, small tubes can be threaded anywhere in the body's arterial system. In Simon's case, a dye will be injected through the catheter into targeted areas, allowing Dr. Heran to obtain detailed images of Simon's spinal blood vessels, all in preparation for the nerve ablation procedure, which is three weeks away.

It's going to be a long day of waiting, especially for Simon, who can't eat anything until after the procedure. But we're old pros at days like these, and we settle into a meditative pace as we move through the various queues and waiting rooms. When Simon is finally settled into his pre-op bed, I dart back to the hotel.

The previous night we left messages of complaint with the manager and then further snitched out Andy by talking to Simon's case worker at WorkSafeBC, Rory, who had made the initial booking with the hotel. After assuring us that he had, of course, booked an accessible room, Rory called the manager, threatening that WorkSafe would take their business elsewhere if official hotel policy for wheelchair-accessible rooms was not clarified to the people working at the front desk. Like magic, an accessible room became available.

Simon's wait time in pre-op is about two hours, which gives me plenty of time to pack up and switch to the new room. When I return, there's still forty-five minutes left before he's scheduled to be wheeled away.

Forty-five minutes stretches to an hour, then two. A nurse tells us there's been a delay due to an emergency. A half hour later Simon and I notice that Dr. Heran has entered the pre-op room and is talking to two women, one younger, one older. A mother and daughter, likely. It's evident even from a distance that a difficult conversation is unfolding, and we try not to stare, or listen. But the three are seated directly in our line of vision, and there is an emotional gravity to their interaction that's hard to turn away from.

Dr. Heran is an interventional radiologist. When I confessed that I had no idea what that meant, he laughed and said even his parents weren't sure what his job description was. He explained that an interventional radiologist treated cases that ran the full spectrum of weird and unusual, specializing in vascular anomalies, blood vessel injuries, and tumors hidden deep in the tissues of the body. He routinely saves lives and has likely done so this very morning.

This, of course, is tremendously impressive. But, in the moment, what impresses me is the compassion in his body language and facial expressions. As he speaks, the older woman cries out, and Dr. Heran places a hand on her shoulder. I hear the word ICU. The word *intubation*. Ten years ago, I had a similar conversation with a trauma doctor. A raw and visceral recognition surges through me and I know, without a doubt, that Dr. Heran's evident kindness is profoundly meaningful.

Shortly after, Dr. Heran arrives at Simon's bedside smiling broadly and apologizing for the delay, assuring us the schedule will get back on track. "It won't be much longer," he says. His relaxed competency is infectious. The usual grumblings of hungry, stressed-out pre-op patients are noticeably absent in this room.

"It's impressive, no?" I say, when Dr. Heran moves on to the next patient. "The way he can start the day with an emergency and then have to pivot to start his *actual* workday by putting a roomful of patients who have been waiting for him for hours at ease."

"He must have nerves of steel," Simon says. "Or, more like nerves of rubber. Something a little livelier."

"Yeah. That's how we need to think about our neuroplastic interventions," I say. "How do we re-rubberize your nervous system? Convince it you're safe?" Until his accident, Simon hadn't had a huge amount of experience with vulnerability. But now, simple things were difficult. Things like showing up at a hotel and being told the accessible room is no longer available, or playing music in relatively inaccessible venues, along with the countless other problems that unexpectedly arise from navigating a world not built for those with mobility issues. "Keeping in mind," I add, "that your nervous system is assessing safety not just within your body, but in the world at large."

"That's a topic likely worth a longer conversation," Si says. The elderly man in the hospital bed beside him moans. Like Simon, he is clothed only in a flimsy blue gown. Deep, cadaverous shadows encircle his partially closed eyes, the bones of his skull prominent under papery skin. He appears to be only minimally conscious. "But maybe not right now."

"Yeah, definitely," I say. "Not right now."

SIMON IS WHEELED into the procedural suite at 1:00. I bustle down to the nearest grocery store, where I spend too much money on comfort foods. At 3:45 a nurse calls: Simon is in the recovery room and he's starving. I return to the hospital pronto, with a latte, a banana, and a blueberry-oatmeal muffin. When I arrive, his nurse, Hazel, is taking his blood pressure. It's high. "I'll be back in ten minutes," she says. "We'll check that blood pressure again, after you've had something to eat."

Simon beams up at me. His face is flushed and, still influenced by the anesthetic drugs, he is pleasantly stoned.

"I never went fully under," he says, taking wolf-bites of muffin. "There was music playing the whole time: Elton John, Pink Floyd, Paul Simon. I was telling Dr. Heran about seeing Paul Simon's final concert."

"Was it weird being awake?"

"No, not really. The only hitch was they tried to go into the right artery, but there was some issue. I don't know what. They switched to the left side." He pulls up his hospital gown, briefly flashing me, so I can see the two insertion sites, each at the middle of the very top of his thighs.

"Well, let's hope those don't leave scars on your bikini line," I say.

Simon grins. "It's a thought that haunts me."

Hazel returns, wrapping the blood pressure cuff around Simon's arm. "Well, look at that," she says. "Almost back to normal. You just needed some food." She smiles at me. Her long, wheat-colored hair is pulled into a tidy twist on top of her head, and she exudes a fine-boned strength. "Or maybe you just needed your wife."

Pulling up the edges of Si's gown, she presses into the skin around the insertion site, first on the right and then on the left, explaining that she'll be doing these checks every ten minutes for the first few hours. Usually recovery time is about two hours, but because Simon is in a wheelchair, his care team wants to double that. "The hip flexion that happens when seated is the worst position after this type of procedure," Hazel explains. "Simon needs to stay lying flat as long as possible. You'll be here until at least eight o'clock."

I make one more trip down to the first floor of the hospital, where I buy another round of warm drinks and a pack of cards. We read our books in Simon's cubicle, and snack, and play several hands of crib. Simon is up three games to my two when Hazel returns to let us know her shift is ending. "Before I go, I want to walk you through what to do if there is a complication after you leave the hospital. It's rare, but they do happen."

"Okay," I say.

"It's a serious issue if the insertion site begins to bulge with blood. See..." she says, pressing into the top of Si's left thigh, "... right now the skin is soft, pliable. Feel it."

I mimic her pressing motion. Under my fingertips, Simon's skin is warm, elastic, alive. "Okay. Got it."

"But if you notice any discoloration, or bruising, or the skin growing taut, that means there is blood pooling. It can happen quickly, so you have to be ready to act fast."

"Okay." My heart sags down toward my gut. I appreciate Hazel's clear, concise instructions. But something in her calm, practical manner is alarming.

"If at any time the skin bruises or bulges, you must immediately apply as much pressure as you can to the top of the surgery site. Like this." She demonstrates by placing her hands, one on top of the other, at the top of Simon's thigh and leaning her full weight in. "No amount of pressure is too much. Hold it for fifteen minutes, and the bulging should subside. Then get into emergency as quickly as possible. But if the bulging doesn't recede with pressure, call 911 right away. Got it?"

I nod. "Got it." From the bed, Simon gives me a wide-eyed, *what-the-fuck* kind of look.

Hazel smiles. "It's an unlikely scenario, but it's best to be prepared."

"Thank you," I say.

Shortly afterward, a new nurse arrives. She's about the same age as Hazel, late twenties, but lacks her warmth. She doesn't introduce herself, and she is aghast that Simon will be leaving the hospital in a wheelchair in under an hour.

"It's not like we have an option," I say. "The hotel is only five minutes away."

"Still," she says. "He shouldn't be in a seated position. Standing or lying down for at least the next twenty-four hours."

"Well, standing is not an option. And we need to travel home tomorrow. That's, minimum, a three-hour trip. Likely longer."

"No, that's not okay." She furrows her brow in a patronizing scowl. "This is *serious.* It's his *femoral artery.*"

"Well, yes," I say. "I get that. But everyone knew he was a wheelchair user. If it is so serious, then you better admit him overnight."

She scowls again. This, obviously, is not an option. "I'm going to make some phone calls."

I take a deep breath before turning back to Simon. "It'll be fine," I say.

"Of course it will."

"First question: Do we walk back, or take the van? Van might be smoother, but I'll need to drop you off at the hotel and then leave you while I return it to the parking lot."

"Walk. It will be fastest. We'll be together the whole time. And it's not any bumpier than getting in and out of the van."

"I could call an accessible taxi," I say.

"And we'd likely wait half an hour for a two-minute ride. Me sitting up the whole time. And I always bounce around in the back of those taxis. No. Walking is best."

The scowling nurse returns with an update. She has consulted with two doctors. The first felt the long trip home tomorrow was reasonable and could be accomplished safely. But the second agreed with the nurse: it would be too long, too soon, in a seated position. She strongly recommends we stay a third night in the hotel room.

My mind lurches. It was hard enough to score the accessible room for tonight. There's no guarantee it will be available for an additional one. "I'll see what I can do."

"This is *serious,*" she says again.

"Right," I say. "You've made that clear." Now, the five blocks from hospital to hotel room seems an impassable distance, a journey as fraught with danger as crossing a minefield. Would a little jostle or curb-bump, or the pain spasm that either might set off, result in dangerous pressure on Simon's fragile femoral arteries? This nurse has succeeded in making me feel suddenly, intensely terrified, and I don't like it. And I can't stop anger from hardening my words. "And again, I have to ask, if it is so serious, then why are you releasing him?"

She returns my tone of obvious frustration with an intensified scowl but doesn't reply.

As eight o'clock approaches, I help Simon dress. Usually he would do this on his own even though it's a tricky maneuver in a tiny hospital bed, requiring a certain amount of bending at the waist, rolling, and throwing of unmoving legs here, then there. That is, strain. Now, I inch each pant leg slowly up, on the right, then the left. This is excruciatingly slow but not particularly stressful, as Simon remains lying down throughout. It's the final stage—getting the pants up over his bum—that I'm dreading. It will require him to sit up for the first time since the procedure and lift his bottom, which in turn will require all the muscles in his torso to tighten.

Simon is unusually silent. I am unusually talkative, maintaining a steady patter of the obvious. *Okay, I'm going to lift your leg here. All right, we've reached your knees. Just a little farther now. Okay, time for the seat lift.* Then it's over. So far so good. But now Simon is upright, in the dangerous seated position, so there's no time to pause. I quickly shove his shoes onto his feet. In the background the nurse hovers. My back is to her, but I can feel the heat of her scowl.

Now comes the real test: the transfer from bed to wheelchair. To accomplish this, Simon must lean forward, deeply creasing the area around the insertion site, and then use momentum to swing his paralyzed hips and legs into the chair: it's a move that requires a certain amount of abandon. This will be the most dangerous step, and one that will necessarily be repeated when we're back at the hotel, alone. My breath catches as Si leans forward to grab the far arm of his wheelchair. He inhales and makes the leap, landing with a thud. For a moment, all three of us stand suspended, waiting to see what will happen.

The nurse moves first. "Okay," she says. "Let's check those insertion sites." The elastic band of Simon's sweatpants is loose and she tugs both sides down, pressing her hands on either side of his groin. "It looks good," she says, her scowl transforming into a face-softening smile.

"Thank you," Simon says, gracious on behalf of us both. I'm not wasting any time on pleasantries and begin pushing the wheelchair before she has a chance to answer. Well wishes or warnings, I don't want to hear any more.

"Okay, babe," I say as we glide toward the exit. "Let's get the hell out of here."

The next twenty-four hours go smoothly. We arrive at the hotel, and Simon transfers into bed, safely returning to a supine position. I secure the room for an additional night without too much hassle. We sleep lightly in the unfamiliar and noisy surroundings, but both of us manage to wake almost two hours later than usual. Our stash of snacks is abundant and ranges from wholesome to decadent: organic cheesy puffs, lemon yogurt, raspberry thumbprint cookies, and various soups and smoothies. The liquid foods are at my insistence: when feeling imperiled, I tend to hydrate. The day passes slowly but not unpleasantly. That is, until seven o'clock that night, when everything goes horribly, terribly wrong.

IT ALL BEGINS with a plan to address Simon's bowel care. Some people are squeamish when it comes to talking about poop, but, post-paralysis, this social convention has become meaningless for us. It's a relentlessly underscored fact of our life that Simon's bowel care requires thought and careful planning. There's no room to be precious. And we've learned—the hard way—that the key to avoiding unwanted accidents is to adhere to a strict schedule. When Si was in rehab, this was repeated like a mantra: *Bowels love routine*. Already Simon's schedule is a day behind. And we're worried that two to three hours of a bowel routine, followed by three to four hours of travel time, is too much to cram into tomorrow morning.

"It's been a full twenty-four hours," Si says. "I think it's best if I break up the seated time: I'll do my bowel routine tonight, get back into bed, and then we leave early tomorrow."

The bathroom is poorly constructed as an accessible space, and apprehension prickles the back of my neck as I watch Simon struggle to maintain his balance on the toilet in the unfamiliar setting. And sure enough, in under ten minutes the skin around the left femoral site grows taut.

"Is it...?" Si says.

"Yes," I say. "You have to get off. Now."

"I can't," Si says. "I've already started my routine. Once it's started, it's started—"

"Now!" I shout. The taut skin has already begun to bulge to the size of an egg. "I'll put down spill pads. It's just poop. We can deal with that. But you need to get off. Now."

"Yeah, yeah," Simon says. "Okay." We are both silent as I help him transfer into his wheelchair and then back into bed. The bulge is now the size of a tomato. I press down with both hands, trying to recall Hazel's clear instructions from the day before. *Press for fifteen minutes until the bulge disappears. Then come into emergency. But if it continues to grow, call 911 immediately.* Despite the pressure of my full weight the bulge morphs into a grotesque and unbelievable size. Apple, I think. Grapefruit.

"We need to call 911," I say. This poses a problem. My cell phone is on the other side of the room. I reach with one hand to the bedside phone and dial down to the front desk. "This is room 612," I shout into the upturned receiver. "I need you to call 911. It's an emergency."

A minute later the manager lets himself into our room, holding a cell phone out so I can give the emergency line operator the pertinent details. She assures us an ambulance will be there shortly and then hangs up.

"I'm sorry," Simon says to the manager. "You've caught me in a very undignified state."

"No, no." The poor man doesn't know where to look and quickly excuses himself to check on the paramedics.

"The ambulance will be here soon," I say.

Simon nods.

Seven more minutes pass. It is an eternity. I'm terrified that Simon's femoral artery will rupture under my hands and he'll bleed out and I won't be able to do anything. We hold each other with our eyes as I continue to lean my full body weight into the ballooning artery, pressing down, holding on, with all my strength.

"It's okay, baby," Simon says. "Breathe. Just breathe."

TWO PARAMEDICS, a man and woman, arrive in a welcome wave of professionalism that sweeps through the private space of our hotel room. Suddenly I'm acutely aware of Simon's nakedness.

"I'm Heather, and this is Danny." They both smile, exuding a lean efficiency. "Okay," Heather says. "Tell us what's happening."

When our synopsis is complete, Danny says, "You've done great, but I'll take over now. We're going to prep Simon for transfer. You have a minute to grab anything you might need. We have to get to the hospital quickly."

"Okay." I step back as Danny takes my spot and Heather checks Simon's vitals. I pull on a pair of jeans, think *purse, Simon's wallet.* My purse is on the floor in the hallway, but when I go to retrieve Simon's wallet, it's not anywhere. Behind me, Simon is apologizing, explaining paralysis and neurogenic bowels. "I had just started my routine and so I'm not sure what will happen now. But if my bowels start to move I won't be able to control it."

"Understood," Heather says.

Double-checking all the spots where Simon's wallet might be, I am filled with an irrational certainty that I have misplaced it. Did I leave it behind in our first hotel room? My hands are shaking. I triple-check, fluttering from one side of the room to the other like a bird flapping its wings against a wall of glass windows.

"It's time to go," Danny says.

When we arrive at the ER, rattling into the crowded waiting area, I'm shocked to see it's only 7:34. Time, like Simon's artery, has ballooned. It was 7:00 when Simon decided to get out of bed. Those seven minutes waiting for the ambulance really were an eternity. There is a sense of cartoonish violence at being thrust back into everyday time and space. This space in particular. The fluorescent lights cast an overexposed glare across the faces of sick and injured people. Another pair of paramedics park a gurney beside us and begin to snap their fingers at the left side of an old woman's face. She's mostly unresponsive, her few attempts at words resembling a gurgling infant pre-language, and her eyes insist on drifting to the right.

"Look here, Audrey. Look over here," the burly paramedic shouts. He continues to snap his fingers in staccato bursts, occasionally alternating them with the sharp report of a hand clap. It is deeply unsettling.

Heather has tucked hospital blankets all around Simon, so he is covered. But the blankets are flimsy and not nearly warm enough for the drafty room. It's hard to see him so vulnerable, especially in an environment that's so abrasive. But Simon, amazing Simon, is smiling and talking hockey with Danny, who continues to apply steady pressure on his left thigh. It's hard to see, but my guess is that the bulge is smaller. More like the size of a baseball.

A nurse with a clipboard introduces herself as Eleanor. She gets an update from the paramedics and then asks Simon and me a few questions. "One last thing," Simon says, as she's about to go. Again he begins with an apology, and then describes his neurogenic bowel. "I can't predict what will happen in the next few hours. I'm so sorry."

She nods with grim professionalism. "Thanks for letting me know. I'm going to get a room set up for you."

At 7:45 Simon is wheeled back into the ER, and we say goodbye to Heather and Danny. A heavy sandbag is placed on Simon's thigh to maintain pressure, and he is deemed stable.

"It's busy tonight," Eleanor says. "It's going to be a wait."

She leaves and we are, abruptly, all alone in a small examination room.

"That was scary," I say, reaching for Si's hand.

"Yeah," he says. "And I really hope I don't take a shit in this bed. Did you bring my meds?"

"Oh no!" I explain how I got hung up looking for his wallet. "I couldn't find it. I kind of lost my mind. Then we had to leave." A new and terrible thought strikes me. "Oh, Beau. I forgot your wheelchair."

"It wouldn't have fit in the ambulance."

"But I didn't even think of it." I'm horrified. It's as if I left a part of Simon's body behind. "I'm so sorry. I should have just wheeled it to the hospital. I likely would have been as fast on foot. I could have met you at the ER." Even as I say it, I know there was no way I would have left Simon's side in that moment.

"No. You needed to be in the ambulance. You can get the chair later."

"Right." I exhale. "We'll see the doctor. Then we'll make a plan."

"Yeah. Now all we can do is wait."

As the hours pass and Simon falls behind on his pain med schedule, he becomes increasingly uncomfortable and uncharacteristically grumpy. He wants me to *do* something. But tucked in the back corner of the room and dozing fitfully, he doesn't see what I see when I poke my head into the hallway. Outside it is bedlam. People sit in chairs lining the narrow hallways among the parked gurneys. A young man who claims to have OD'd and then changed his mind paces while loudly complaining about the overhead lights. An old woman yells at him to sit down and shut up. Down the hall, someone coughs, a wet, crackling noise that continues for hours. Right outside our door, a middle-aged woman with long, straight black hair and the misleading plump, rosy cheeks of a chemo patient throws up into a pan, over and over and over again. How uncomfortable she must be, I think, sick and sitting for hours in a rigid plastic chair.

It is a parade of pain that takes my breath away.

I've yet to see a doctor, but the nurses stride by, determinedly avoiding eye contact. As the hallway continues to fill up—a man who thinks he is having a stroke; an old woman, surrounded by family members, wailing in Cantonese—I realize how lucky we are to have a room.

There's not a lot to recommend the threat of incontinence, but I am grateful it has secured us this oasis of privacy.

A doctor arrives just after one o'clock in the morning. She introduces herself, but my tired brain immediately forgets her name, focusing instead on a series of extraneous details: she is left-handed, athletic, impossibly young to so confidently take charge amid all of this mayhem. Behind large black-framed glasses, her eyes are rimmed with dark liner and various shades of shadow, lending a strange and incongruous glamour to her practical face. She reminds me of a fierce Zooey Deschanel. "Simon's situation is potentially very serious," she says. "We'll get some blood work and convince someone at radiology that we need imaging done right away." She smiles apologetically. "'Right away' might still be a bit of a wait."

"Will I have time to run back to the hotel and get Simon's wheelchair?" I ask. "I can get there and back in half an hour."

"Absolutely," she says.

I'm uneasy at leaving Simon unattended in his private room; the nurses would have no idea if things went sideways. The last time we saw Eleanor, our only other in-person contact, was more than five hours ago. But he needs his chair, and so I head to the hotel. Simon's wallet is in the pocket of his satchel. It's a little deeper than usual but by no means hidden. How could I not have seen it? I looked in that pocket *three* times. Animal panic really had temporarily blinded me. Now, I shake my head, shimmy my shoulders, and exhale, trying to shiver the stress out, the way an animal would. It's a TACKLING PAIN tip I read, where I can't remember in the moment. It helps, maybe, even if just as a physical reminder to slow and deepen my breath. With a pack of cards, books, clothes, meds, and wallet balanced in the seat of the wheelchair, I jog back to the hospital, following the late-night route I took so many years ago when Simon was fighting for his life in the ICU.

Tonight, a wet fog is visible in the hazy glow of the street lamps, the stars overhead stifled by damp clouds. The usual busy blur of cars and pedestrians and bikes whizzing past on the narrow streets is stilled at this hour, and, in that stillness, all my senses prick and bristle, extra awake. A squirrel with an oversized corner of bread crust wedged into his pudgy cheeks darts past, skittering up and across a bike stand to disappear into the shadow recesses of an oak tree.

At the ER entrance, a grizzled old guy pulling an IV pole pushes past me, lighting his cigarette even before he's cleared the automatic doors. In the waiting room one of the overhead lights is humming, an insect quiver, as if fireflies and not electricity were powering the bright bulb. It's agitating, adding to my impatience as I wait several long minutes for a nurse to buzz me in.

Now that it is almost 2:00 AM, the deepest gully of the night, the ER hallway is less crowded. A nurse delivers a sandwich and juice to a man who appears to be one of Vancouver's many unhoused citizens. He tears open the cellophane wrapping, then drapes a blanket over his head, covering his face as he eats. Simon is dozing in his brightly lit room, and so I tiptoe to a chair and open my book. But his nap is cut short when a technician clatters in to take his blood. Shortly after that we shuffle down to the radiology department, where Simon undergoes a CT scan. Then back to the ER. The kind of eerie and brittle clarity that comes with a sleepless night descends.

The doctor returns with results. The sudden swelling was caused by a pseudoaneurysm, a collection of blood pooling in the outer membranes of the artery.

"So... how serious is that?" I ask. "What's the chance a pseudoaneurysm becomes a real aneurysm?"

She shrugs, palms open. Who knows? "I've requested a vascular surgeon consult. He should be here shortly." Her sudden grin is mischievous, and again I'm struck with her resemblance to Zooey Deschanel. "I woke him up!"

The vascular surgeon arrives, bike helmet in hand, and introduces himself as Alexander. He's young and says *fair enough* repeatedly as Simon, loquacious with lack of sleep, describes the night's events. Alexander compliments him for being a good storyteller. An extended, awkward pause follows, broken when Alexander clears his throat. "The scan results were not definitive," he says. "But often these pseudoaneurysms heal on their own. Right now, there is no clear reason for a surgical intervention. So, you're free to be discharged. But we'd like to do a repeat scan in a week."

He leaves, and we let the news sink in. Simon is relieved. I am too, of course. But the prospect of discharge is also terrifying. It is 4:15 in the morning.

"What do we do next?" I say. "Should we book the hotel room for the week, until the next scan? Stay close to the hospital?"

"No," Simon says. "So far, bowel-wise, I've been lucky. But I need my bathroom. If we leave now we can catch the first ferry. Traffic won't be bad. We'll be home by mid-morning."

A four-hour trip with Simon seated the whole way? It feels impossibly dangerous. "Si, I don't—"

"Stan. I *need* to be home."

"Okay," I say. "I hear you." We buy two espressos, rub our bleary eyes, and head out, thankfully making it all the way back home without any further drama.

BRUISES LIKE THUNDERCLOUDS erupt in magnificent billows of plum, gunmetal gray, and indigo across Simon's thighs and groin. My heart stutters every time he reaches for a cup or plate creasing at his hips to lean forward. After a tense week of waiting, we return to Vancouver General Hospital for the check-up scan. The news is good. The pseudo-aneurysm has healed on its own, and the nerve ablation can proceed as planned.

# 11

# Be Easy, Bruv

MARCH 22, DAY 243.
*Twelve days before the nerve ablation procedure.*

DESPITE OUR GREAT RELIEF, I continue to relive those terrifying moments in the hotel room and the anxious hours that followed. Simon admits the episode lingers for him too. The thought of returning to the hospital in less than two weeks for the nerve ablation procedure fills us both with dread.

"I'm sorry," Simon says. "Dealing with my stupid body is a full-time job."

"And the pay is shit," I say.

"C'mon now," he says. "There's a few perks. I'll make you Caesar salad and homemade sourdough pizza tonight."

So, this is how we cope: we take a weekend off from talking, or thinking, about pain. When it flares, Simon pops an extra hydromorphone and we do our best to ignore it. We eat comfort food in front of the TV, binge-watching the new season of *Fleabag*.

By Monday we're sufficiently restored to call an impromptu TACKLING PAIN meeting to assess the strategies from the *Neuroplastic Transformation* workbook. Some have helped, and we'll continue to use them. Often in the middle of the night, Simon will request that I restart the diffuser filled with peppermint oil or play the recording of the Tibetan singing bowls.

And although our attempt at sign language failed, Simon has made his own adaption, tapping his thumb to each finger in sequence, back and forth, and breathing deeply, like a yogi. We figure his musician's fingers must have cornered enough cortical real estate that tactilely stimulating them might be effective in countering the flares of pain. We've even developed a few joke strategies. Sometimes Simon shouts like Gandalf to the Balrog demon in *Lord of the Rings*: "Pain, you shall not pass!" Other times, he inhales deeply and says in his best Trump voice, "Fake news, this is just fake news." Overall the neuroplastic strategies have been most helpful in prompting us to be more active and creative in how we approach his pain.

Still, some of Simon's skepticism remains. "The workbook puts a fancy name to a basic strategy: attempt to consciously distract yourself," he says. "Sometimes I think these interventions are the equivalent of turning up a car radio so you don't hear that ominous clanking in your engine. The kind of clanking you ignore at your peril."

So we've expanded our research to include the Explain Pain series, which consists of three books, each rated for the density of medical language. Today Simon is reading *The Explain Pain Handbook: Protectometer.* It's designed as an interactive workbook for those with chronic pain and rates somewhere between *almost none* and *a bit* on the Scientific Jargon Meter. I am reading *Explain Pain,* which is intended for clinicians, patients, and anyone interested in pain science, and hovers midway on the meter. There is also *Explain Pain Supercharged*, which has the highest rating, and a companion to the series, *Painful Yarns,* which has the lowest.

The latter is a collection of playful tales that illustrate key principles of pain science. I was delighted when I read the first story, as it was basically an elaborate version of Simon's turning-up-the-car-radio-to-drown-out-the-sounds-of-engine-trouble analogy. Maybe, at last, we've found pain scientists who (metaphorically) speak his language.

The books cite the most up-to-date research and contain an extensive list of further references. It's impressive. Like so many other resources, the Explain Pain series starts with the challenging premise that all pain is created in the brain, without exception. The introductory section of the book stresses the highly contextual nature of pain: the same minor finger injury will produce more pain in the brain of a professional violinist than in the brain of a professional dancer because a finger injury more directly threatens the violinist's identity and livelihood. Authors Lorimer Moseley and David Butler build from the premise that when pain persists, especially for no known reason, it is a *biopsychosocial* experience, jeopardizing everything from a person's physical well-being and ease in the world to their self-identity, their job and housing security, and their most important relationships. This overarching sense of threat, Moseley and Butler tell us, contributes directly to the pain experience: your body is working *too* hard to protect you. Their research demonstrates that people are empowered to reduce threat levels when they know what's occurring within their bodies. Understanding the biology of pain removes some of its uncertainty, and this is important because uncertainty, and the stress it can cause, exacerbates pain.

Butler and Moseley resist defining chronic pain as a disease, instead recommending that chronic pain sufferers identify their DIMs—Dangers in Me—basically, any factors that pose a credible threat. This might be something tangible, like a knee joint that has inexplicably swollen to twice its usual size, or a radiology report peppered with alarming words like *degeneration* or *atrophy.* But it might also be something less tangible, such as an insistent, catastrophizing belief that you're destined to live with severe mobility issues. It might even be something as seemingly unrelated as a dizzying rise in interest rates. Your ability to work full-time has been compromised because of pain. What if you can't manage a ballooning mortgage payment? Will you lose your house?

To counter a list of DIMs, Moseley and Butler suggest making a second list of SIMs, or Safety in Me, again spanning a broad range of biological, psychological, and social factors. A marked improvement in health might be a SIM, but so might a health care practitioner's acknowledgment that your pain is real and complex, or a close friend showing up unexpectedly with takeout Thai food.

If a credible sense of safety outweighs the credible threat of danger, Moseley and Butler argue, there's a good chance that the hypervigilance of chronic pain states will be reduced, and that pain will once more be returned to its important evolutionary role as an early warning system for danger. Expanding *neuroplastic* to *bioplastic,* they assure the reader that all of the systems of the body—not just the brain—are changeable and adaptable.

"Listen to this," I say to Simon, reading out loud from my book:

> We believe that all pain experiences are normal and are an excellent, though unpleasant, response to what your brain judges to be a threatening situation. We believe

> that even if problems do exist in your joints, muscles, ligaments, nerves, immune system or anywhere else, it won't hurt if your brain thinks you are not in danger. In exactly the same way, even if no problems whatsoever exist in your body tissues, nerves or immune system, it will still hurt if your brain thinks you are in danger. It is as simple and as difficult as that.

"Hhhmpf," Si grunts. "*Unpleasant*. That's a word."

It is. I'm realizing it's the go-to euphemism for pain scientists and clinicians. *Unpleasant.* Such a bland word to describe the messy, frayed, horrifying dissolution of self that accompanies persistent pain. Simon can't help but feel that it diminishes the reality of what he lives with daily. He can't help but feel that the person using that word simply doesn't get it. And maybe that is the case. *Explain Pain* specifically states at the outset that as a guidebook it's especially suited to people who experience chronic non-specific pain, like the kind of low back pain that troubled me for years. A book like this would have been helpful when I was working through pain that lasted off and on over a decade and was both difficult and unpleasant. But would it work for Simon?

It's a thought to return to later. But in the moment, I can't help but feel relief. At a certain point, it had been important to think of Simon's pain as a chronic disease simply so that we could move out of a constant state of emergency. When the pain surged through his body, we had to retrain ourselves to ignore the impulse to scream, SOMETHING'S WRONG! DO SOMETHING. RIGHT NOW!

But even then I believed that Simon's body had a strong impulse toward healing. Because of paralysis, there was a blaring sensory and motor silence below his waist. Each time his nervous system checked in and discovered that disturbing silence—a major biological DIM—his brain concluded something was wrong. More healing was required. Further action was needed. There was something comforting in returning to the notion that pain—even if it was part of a misfiring, hypervigilant system—was still a deep expression of the body's need for wholeness, balance, and safety.

"The word *unpleasant* aside, it's an interesting way to approach pain, don't you think?" I ask.

"Yeah," he says, unconvincingly. "But the kind of things they list as DIMS don't apply to me, really, and my SIMS, things like having a supportive spouse, family, community, and medical team, are all in place. Apparently the fear of ending up in a wheelchair is a major DIM, and I'm already there, so whatever. It's pain that's my main DIM, and so is bowel and bladder care. Playing music is both a DIM and a SIM, I think. I love it but it stresses me out. Thing is, I'm pretty sure I have way more SIMS than DIMS, so by this equation I shouldn't be in pain."

"So—do you find the *Protectometer* goofy?"

"Well. Yes. And no. I appreciate that they're keeping it straightforward. And... lighthearted. My pain-addled brain couldn't tackle the density of the book you're reading. At least not right now. But these?" He pulls open a foldout section of the book that contains a row of rainbow sticky notes meant for him to create his own colorful DIM and SIM list. "Let's just say quirky office supply accoutrements don't excite me the way they do you."

"Fair. But, listen. Given the current surplus of post-angiogram, post-aneurysm, pre-ablation DIMS we're both experiencing, I think we should take the next few days to be extra kind to ourselves. Buy takeout. Find another binge-worthy series. Lie low. Reduce expectations."

"In other words: *Be easy, bruv,*" Si says in a British accent. It's a line from a BBC cop drama we watched recently.

"Yeah," I say. "Be easy."

THE NEXT DAY DAWNS OVERCAST. Rain, then fog, then a determined west wind that sends the clouds skittering like dust bunnies to the far corners of the horizon. By mid-afternoon the sky is a jeweled blue and the sun is shining. After so many wet, gray days it's a welcome reprieve, and I convince Simon to come for a walk in the forest. The Sunshine Coast is a narrow spit of land sandwiched between the sea and mountains. But although there are trees and trails everywhere, the only well-maintained, fully wheelchair-accessible path is a twenty-five-minute drive away. As we pull into the Hidden Grove parking lot, Chico lets out an extended whine of anticipation.

Over the past ten years the phrase *quality of life* had, like *neuroplasticity,* become ubiquitous in our world. When Simon was in a coma in the ICU, I was told that medical decisions would be based on his potential for *quality of life.* Later, rehab protocols were built around what would provide Simon with the best *quality of life.* And when applying for funding, say, to build wheelchair-accessible garden beds, we had learned how important it was to emphasize how this new project would improve his *quality of life.* Before his accident, though, we—like most people—had never given explicit thought to the notion of *quality of life.* If pressed, we might have said that the foundation for any kind of quality of life was good health.

But what is good health when "all better" is not an option? The singular event of Si's accident, and all the rippling consequences, had provided us with ample opportunity to question all our previously held beliefs. Healthy people tend to take their health for granted. Certainly we did. Health, for the healthy, is a given, a natural state; this is the innocently arrogant viewpoint held by those who have never yet felt betrayed by their body.

For Simon, health has become a moving target, a relative goal. Where once health had meant the absence of illness, or injury, now it means something different—resilience, maybe? A general sense of equilibrium and balance? Paralysis in his legs and left side means that Simon struggles to maintain his physical balance, even seated, but he can cultivate balance in other areas of his life, in his intellectual and artistic pursuits and in his many roles—as a father, husband, son, friend, and musician. He can wake up strong enough to tackle another difficult day. But pain, that great disruptor, constantly undermines his resilience and balance. It takes a much greater conscious effort to plan and execute "relaxing activities," and our perspective on these types of activities has undergone a seismic shift. No longer do we consider them an indulgent luxury or even a well-earned reward at the end of a busy work week. Now they are a critical part of his recovery.

It's an uphill roll across the gravel parking lot, and both Simon and I are out of breath even before we reach the trailhead.

"Thanks for the assist," Simon says, panting.

"Yeah, well, I'm not sure relaxing should be so much work," I say, also panting.

"Right? I think Sisyphus had greater ambitions for his

boulder," Si says, "than just having a few hours of fun down time."

"Yep."

In the forest, the path evens out. The world breathes a luminous green, and we're immediately drenched in leafy incandescence, the air suffused with phytoncides, the health-inducing organic compounds released by the trees. The Japanese practice of *shinrin-yoku,* or forest bathing, is a kind of contemplative communion with the natural world. And that's exactly how I feel entering this cathedral of old-growth trees: showered in emerald, jade, sea-green.

I love it here.

Simon's health issues are often so pressing and generally command so much of our joint focus, it's easy to forget that I need rebalancing time too. But when things go all to hell, as they did last week, this is the place that helps to restore my equanimity. Most often I come here with Chico, a brief respite from the demands (or allostatic stressors) of my life, but I'm glad Simon's here today and tell him so.

"Thanks. I know it means more work for you, and you don't actually get the long hike you want." He points at my Fitbit. "You won't get your steps in today."

"Ha! Chico and I can do that tomorrow," I say. "Plus, it's nice being in the forest moving slow, hanging out. It's a different kind of experience."

"It's big of you to say that, Stan. I know how important those steps are."

He's teasing me for my single-minded devotion to a ten-thousand-step day. But it's a loving tease, because he also knows that regular exercise is a cornerstone of my sanity, and that, sometimes, setting small, achievable goals—like ten thousand steps—in the midst of chaos can be an important gesture of self-care.

Radically slowing down isn't always an easy or comfortable thing to do, something we both learned firsthand in the years after his accident. At first, it was a terrifying sensation in which both of us felt untethered from the reassuring structure of ordinary, busy, everyday life. Simon compared it to being an astronaut, floating in space. No lifeline; no ship.

But in the intervening years we've built our own lifelines, the small gestures and regular routines that rescue us in times of great anxiety or grief. Most of these routines involve either movement or music, sometimes both. And food. Both of us are opportunistic omnivores; even in the toughest times, we like to eat.

We've had to work to balance health concerns with overall pleasure. "Diets, schmiets" is Simon's general position when it comes to nutritional plans. (He also teases me for my willingness to embrace the latest superfood craze and my susceptibility to marketing campaigns. "Amaranth?" he said once, in response to my suggesting an alternative to his beloved basmati rice. "Is that one of the *ancient* grains?") But now, he readily admits a cavalier attitude toward nutrition is no longer one he can sustain, and over the past few years we have at times, in response to various health crises, made radical changes, ultimately settling on a diet that follows general anti-inflammatory rules: increase good fats, leafy greens, and nutrient-dense, plant-based foods; reduce simple carbohydrates, processed food, and sugary treats; opt, when possible, for foods that are local and seasonal. But neither of us is ascetic by nature, and there's joy to be found in the occasional indulgence. Paralysis means that many of life's simple, sensual pleasures are not readily available to Simon. The acts of planning and preparing food and the togetherness of enjoying a good meal are also top priorities; the *how* and *why* of eating are as important as what we consume.

Simon is in charge of bringing the music. Both before and after his accident he has always—but especially in times of great need—filled our home with communal laughter and song. For him, it's exercise, or some kind of restorative movement practice, that has been tough. We both know he needs a supportive plan to gradually increase his physical activity, but somehow knowing that doesn't make it any easier to put in place.

"I know more exercise would eventually make me feel better," Si says. "But I hate the way it makes me have to face up to my physical limitations. It makes me sad. And being sad makes me mad. And I hate being mad. It's a lot of sad-mad-hate to go through before you get to the good stuff."

I nod. "Let's leave off discussing exercise for now. Remember: it's a week of low expectations. Be easy, bruv."

The trail circles around an uprooted cedar. Up ahead, golden sheaves of sunshine slant through the broad arms of the trees, pooling in the ferny undergrowth. Chico darts through the splashes of light, sniffing moss-covered stumps and chasing squirrels. Simon smiles as he leans into rolling up a slight incline. "You're right. Let's talk dinner. An abundance of fish tacos might be the only thing to heal the horror of last week and manage the anticipation of the week to come."

"Salmon?"

"No. Cod."

"Garlic aioli? Or cilantro pesto?"

"Desperate times call for desperate measures," Simon says. "We definitely need both."

# 12

# Broken Healing

APRIL 3, DAY 255.
*The night before the nerve ablation procedure.*

"CHECK IT OUT," I say. "It's a virtual reality arcade." It's spring in Vancouver. Tiny banks of cherry blossoms edge the double-wide storefront, the one-way glass lit with an early evening glow. The air is warm. After months of cold rain, it's so flagrantly lovely outside that we've decided to walk, and wheel, to our dinner date. Our son, Eli, knowing how nervous we are about the nerve ablation procedure tomorrow, has insisted on treating us to a meal at a fancy Italian restaurant. It's been a pleasure to walk, but the route is longer and steeper than we anticipated, and Simon has required a push assist.

"Very different from the arcades when we were kids, hey?" Simon says. "The world has moved way past *Frogger* and *Arkanoid*."

"No kidding," I say, suddenly breathless. We've hit a section of sharp incline, and wordlessly Simon and I combine efforts: I push as he wheels furiously all the way to the top of the hill, where the restaurant awaits.

Dinner is divine. Eli introduces us to Emma, his new girlfriend. My quick eye contact with Simon as the appetizers are served confirms that he shares my initial impression:

this is a serious relationship. It's evident in their easy, connected body language. We tuck into plates of ash-roasted beets and homemade ravioli as Eli refills our wineglasses. The conversation veers wildly, from the gritty play of the Raptors to Marc Rebillet's upcoming tour dates to the latest news in robotic exoskeletons designed for the paralyzed to the current programs at the Vancouver Aquarium, where Emma works.

The sun has gone down by the end of the delicious four-course meal, but it's still warm outside, the air laced with the scent of lilac. We decide not to call a taxi but to walk back the way we came.

"The return trip will be more downhill," Si says. "Easy peasy."

"Are you guys sure?" Eli asks. "I can drive you back."

"Thanks, but no," Simon says. "We never get the chance to be out in the city at night. I miss it."

We hug Emma, then Eli. "Call if you need back-up tomorrow," my tall son says, kissing my forehead.

"Thanks, kiddo," Si says. "But this procedure should be straightforward."

"Yeah," I concur. "Straightforward." As if by saying this together we can will it to be so.

On the way back to the hotel we pass the VR arcade again. A lightning bolt of a thought strikes.

"An affordable robotic exoskeleton to get you up walking might be a long way off, but what about using VR technology to create the illusion of movement? As a possible way of treating pain in spinal cord patients?" I say. I'm imagining something similar to what V. S. Ramachandran did with the mirror box for people with phantom limb pain. The more time people engaged with the visual illusion of a fully restored limb, the greater the chance they could address some of their phantom's issues, including pain.

"So how would it work?" Si asks. "I'd see myself walking in the virtual world?"

"Well, I don't know. I don't know anything about the technology, really. But I think it would be best to start small. Like having an avatar seated in a room and when you imagine lifting a knee, the avatar's leg moves. Then maybe you progress through basic functional movements, practicing crawling, opposite hand and knee moving together, working your way to standing, walking, running."

"We could go for a virtual jog together," Si says.

We pass an older man in a hospital-issue wheelchair moving awkwardly down the street. Underdressed in a stained and torn Canucks jersey, he propels the chair by taking tiny steps with his left foot. His right pant leg is twisted into a knot, the leg below the knee missing. Simon nods, but the man ignores him. "Can you imagine if it was part of rehab?" I continue, excited. "If along with your regular physio, you did a few hours of virtual movement as a kind of nervous system reset. A pain prevention protocol."

"It would be tough psychologically," Si says. "Back in rehab, it was hard enough reckoning with the permanence of the injury. But if I had started hanging out in a virtual world where I could go for a walk, or a run, or, you know, play soccer with a virtual Messi, or hoops with LeBron? I would never have wanted to leave."

"Good point," I say. "It could make that transition harder. But imagine if it could be a regular part of your day now. Like, the way somebody else might jog or swim or hike three or four times a week to stay healthy. I mean, if it helped to prevent chronic pain? So what if it hijacks some of your real-world interactions? Pain hijacks your life every day. There's no real risk, like there are with meds or procedures. It's not like you'll end up with a pseudoaneurysm, even if you are in a deadly battle with goblins or Nazis or whomever it is the virtual world is battling these days."

"Well, as you know, I'm more of a lover than a fighter."

"Got it. Forget vanquishing orcs and fascists," I say as we enter the hotel lobby; smug-faced Andy is there behind the check-in counter. "And snooty hotel clerks. Bring on the VR vixens."

"That's it," Si says, as we roll into an empty elevator. "The fully consenting, totally empowered, kick-ass vixens. Bring 'em on."

AFTER THE GOOD MEAL and long walk, Simon falls into an early and unusually deep sleep. But there is a commotion in the adjacent hotel room and I lie awake, restless, an unwilling eavesdropper to ugly, angry words. *Fuck off, leave me alone. Shut the fuck up and act like a fucking adult. Fucking bitch.* I identify four distinct voices, two men, two women. It is a family, maybe, parents and their two nearly grown kids. They are very unhappy. The noises escalate, but then a door slams and the room falls quiet.

Still, I can't sleep. I'm thinking about Patrick Wall's injunction to view pain as a need state, like hunger or thirst. Action needs to be taken to address that need. Wall outlines three appropriate responses to pain. First, distance yourself from harmful stimuli. If your hand is on a hot burner, pull it away. If a shark is snacking on you, get out of the water. Second, adopt a posture to limit further injury and maximize recovery. If your ankle is sprained, elevate it. If you suspect you have injured vertebrae or a brain injury, stop moving and stabilize your spine and head. Third, seek safety, relief, and cure. Pop a few ibuprofens until the swelling in your ankle subsides; complete the full course of antibiotics and rest up until the shark bite heals; or, as was the case for Simon, undergo hours of brain and spinal surgery, reside in an induced coma until your system stabilizes, then spend three to six months in intense rehabilitation.

It strikes me that Wall should have included a final step: a graduated return to movement, because it's always the restoration of functional mobility that convinces our brains that we've finally healed.

This final step would, of course, be complicated if the outcome of an injury was paralysis. For most people who have survived a spinal cord injury, the onset of neuropathic pain is anywhere from three months to a year after the injury. That the onset isn't always immediate is one of the more mysterious aspects of the phenomenon of pain in paralyzed limbs. Why did the pain begin, as it had for Simon, around three months post-accident, roughly when the maximum amount of tissue healing had already occurred? It never made sense. But what if it's as simple as the fact that that final step—movement—in the body's necessary healing sequence is being thwarted? The sequence is frustrated, stuck in a loop that over time results in the escalating experience of persistent pain.

Could virtual reality movement convince a nervous system coping with paralysis that the healing sequence had been satisfied? My brain is busy with these thoughts right up until the moment when I fall into a sound sleep. A few hours later I'm awakened by screams. It's not Simon, although I can tell by his breath he's awake beside me. It's the room next door. Four voices mingle in rage and despair. *Fuck off, you fucking skank. You two are fucking retards. I'm sorry for being fucking alive.*

"Whoa," Simon says.

"It's bad," I say. "Do you think we should call down to the front desk?"

"Nobody sounds like they're getting beaten up, right?"

"No."

"It's hard to see how a hotel clerk, or the cops, are going to make that situation better."

"No. Only worse." We lie still listening. *You are a fucking dog, fuck off. Fuck off! Fuck. Off.*

A fierce, strangulating pain warps and distorts the voices next door. Somewhere, somehow, a healing sequence was broken there too. We lie quietly. Simon slowly softens, his breath lengthening, returning to its usual sleepy purr. The cries in the next room also settle and I drift off, dreams tense and crowded with upset voices, for the last hour before our predawn alarm.

We arrive early at the hospital. Once again, Simon is on a no-food, no-drink protocol, and his stomach gurgles cantankerously as he dons the blue hospital gown. This time, thankfully, there are no delays, and he's wheeled into the procedural suite right on schedule. We're both excited. This is the moment of truth. Will the pain be gone when Simon wakes?

THE PROCEDURE IS taking longer than anticipated—it's almost two hours past the time Simon was meant to be in the recovery room. That I am back in the same hallways and cafeteria and waiting rooms where I lived ten years ago while Simon was in a coma does nothing to stem my growing panic. I call Simon's sister, Emily, who, along with Simon and Eli, is my most trusted ally in times of trouble. She's in Toronto, three hours ahead, nearing the end of her own challenging day, and yet she puts everything aside so that I can rant and catastrophize and reel myself in, then start all over again. This continues for about forty minutes, until a nurse interrupts the call to inform me that Simon is waking from the general anesthetic.

In the recovery room, he is still half-asleep, his face soft and slack until I reach for his hand. A drowsy smile emerges first, Cheshire Cat-like, before he slowly opens weighted eyelids.

"So?" I say. "The pain. Is it gone?"

His shakes his head, knocking the pillow edges framing his face. "No," he says. "But, maybe, muted. A little?" I squeeze his hand, and he closes his eyes and naps for another ten minutes.

Later, on the walk back to the hotel room, Simon reports that the jostles from the bumpy cement aren't setting off spikes of pain the way they usually do. This seems like monumental progress, and our cautious hearts allow a little excited hope to percolate. No pain spike is a good start, and, who knows, maybe it will be even better tomorrow.

But it isn't.

Things get bad on the drive home. Really bad.

I glance in the rearview mirror to where Simon is seated in his wheelchair, anchored by a system of hooks and pulleys to the floor of the van. It's rare for him to ride this way; he loves to drive and usually prefers to transfer into the driver's seat, which is fitted with hand controls. But not today. The pain is so random, volatile, and explosive that he's asked me to take the wheel.

Behind me I hear the catch in his breath and sense him tensing up, and I too tense, bracing myself for his pain cry, which in the next breath fills the van, a merciless unraveling, language dissolving into shrill syllables. The sound rings inside my bones. Simon's face, neck, and torso tremble with tension.

And then a pause. Despite the quiet, the air in the van remains discordant, troubled. As I listen to the effort Simon makes to slow and deepen his breath, my own gnarled muscles slightly release. In the rearview mirror, Simon white-knuckles the overhead hand grips, an ashy paleness clouding his face. His eyes, meeting mine in the mirror, glitter with a febrile shine. He looks like a carsick kid who has gone around one bend too many. Then we drive over a speed bump, and the screaming storm returns.

It is a long trip home.

Not only is the pain still there, but over the next few days, it becomes significantly worse. Much worse than it was pre-procedure. The pain is so bad that Simon can't get out of bed. "I consider myself a pretty upbeat guy," he says, when I bring him a cup of coffee. "But I think I'm depressed."

Dr. Heran emails for an update and Simon asks if I can respond. "I wish we could give him better news," he says. "I feel like I've failed the procedure."

Dr. Heran is equally dismayed. He calls so that the three of us can have a longer conversation. He once again explains that an ablation procedure—in Simon's case, the burning of the dorsal root ganglion—can be accomplished with either extreme heat or extreme cold. For Simon's procedure, heat was used on the right side, cold on the left. Dr. Heran suspects the use of heat has caused increased irritation in the area, but that it should subside in a few weeks. "Let's talk in ten days. Hopefully things will be better. If not, we might want to consider a nerve block."

"We're leaving to visit my parents in Quebec in three weeks," Simon says. "And I'll be there for over a month. Do you think you would be able to squeeze me in for a nerve block before we leave?"

"Absolutely," Dr. Heran says. "We'll make time."

Over the next few days the pain reaches staggering heights. We enter a mourning period. Simon unplugs the phone. I cancel a much-anticipated dinner invitation. We move slowly and quietly and kindly through the days and nights, as if slowness, quietness, and kindness can combat the devastation we both feel. After about two weeks, as Dr. Heran predicted, the pain eases back to pre-ablation levels, and life, more or less, returns to normal.

Simon has had a nerve block three times before with tenuous results. Only one of those three times, it seemed—*maybe*—that his pain was reduced for a couple of weeks afterward. Still, he's keen to have one again. Dr. Heran juggles his jam-packed schedule and Simon books the procedure for two days before we're set to fly to Quebec.

I'm not happy with Simon's new plan. Each of the previous three times, the nerve block procedure has substantially increased Simon's pain for the first ten to fourteen days while the spinal nerves recover from being jabbed by a needle, a possible consequence we had been consistently warned to expect.

"That means increased pain while you're on the five-hour flight east," I say. "And can you really handle another *increase* in pain right now? While we're traveling out of province? I think we need to press pause and wait. Take some time to reassess."

Reluctantly, Simon agrees. It breaks my heart, and I almost wish he would come up with a strong counter-argument. But after all our TACKLING PAIN efforts, neither of us can shake this sense of overwhelming defeat. For the moment, we're done. Simon calls Dr. Heran's office and cancels the appointment.

# 13

# Insider Info

MAY 2, DAY 284.

A shimmering carpet of bluebells spreads across the front yard of Simon's childhood home. This morning we woke to a cloud of geese lifting from the back field, and now goldfinches bustle between the bird feeder on the covered porch and the fuzzy yellow blossoms of the forsythia bush. Over the years our visits with Simon's parents, Marc and Lorna, have usually corresponded with either summer or winter holidays, and so we've rarely experienced this springtime splendor.

Simon will stay here while I fly on to England to attend the International Association for the Study of Pain neuropathic pain conference. Thankfully the week we've spent together here has been restorative. We've slid into his parents' daily routines—slow mornings, afternoon gardening, a bocce-in-the-backyard happy hour, dinner at seven. The stress of the past month has eased, dissolving into the damp spring air.

Unfortunately, this isn't true of Si's pain. Sitting at the sunny breakfast table with his parents, I listen as Simon, rising from bed, is caught in an electric squall of firing nerves. From the bedroom, his cries modulate from holler to scream to breathless whimper. I am mostly numb to these unsettling sounds, but it's upsetting to Simon's parents, who look at each other, then look at me.

"What can we do to help him," Lorna asks, "while you're gone?"

"Nothing that you haven't already done," I say.

This is profoundly true. In the aftermath of Si's accident, his family have supported us in countless big and small ways. While I'm gone, time at the farmhouse will pass in a predictable manner: gentle days filled with animated conversations that dart between the topics of politics, music, sports, and the evening's dinner menu. Simon and his mom will vie for online Scrabble supremacy. At six o'clock or so, Simon and his dad will pick up their guitars and play songs in the living room. After dinner, they'll eat Häagen-Dazs bars and watch the NBA playoffs. Both Si and his father have high hopes the Raptors will go deep this year. Just as he was as a child, Simon will be loved, supported, and nurtured. As much as anything we've done over the past nine months, this visit feels like a critically necessary pain intervention strategy.

"He needs a little extra space in his day," I say now to Simon's mother. "To let the pain move through."

"What?" Simon says, wheeling into the room. He looks back and forth between his parents' stricken faces.

"We're talking about your pain," I say.

"Don't sweat it, it's just fake news," Simon says, wheeling over to the coffee pot. "But... sorry about that, guys. I know it's unpleasant to hear."

"Couldn't the doctor cut the nerves a little higher in the spinal cord?" Simon's mom asks, still desperately reluctant to let go of the hope proffered by the nerve ablation procedure.

"No, Mom." Si loads up the toaster and takes a slurp of coffee. "I might do another nerve block, but I'm done with the ablation."

"The sensitization of Simon's nervous system means there are changes in pain-processing areas all the way up the spinal cord and into the brain," I add, hearing how annoyingly like a pain textbook I sound. "The dorsal root ganglion is a kind of master switch, but if that doesn't work, and it didn't, we can't keep burning nerves higher and higher up."

"Can't they go into the spot in the brain and burn that away?"

"What?" Simon says, laughing. "You mean like a lobotomy, Mom? I've had enough tinkering in my brain."

"And there's not just one spot in the brain. There's a bunch," I say. "But they actually have done lobotomies for pain in the past. Patients still feel pain afterward, but it doesn't bother them one way or another. It's like, 'Pain? Meh!'"

"Because they have lobotomies!" Si says. "Nothing much will bug them ever again. As much as it sucks, I'll take my pain, thanks."

"Okay, okay," Lorna says, still not entirely convinced.

A few days later, Marc and Simon drive me to the airport.

"Write me," Si says when I kiss him goodbye. "Every day. Okay?"

My flight is a red-eye, crammed with businessmen and fussy babies. The young woman beside me is an ideal seatmate: earbuds in, black eye mask on, she is perfectly still the whole six-plus hours. She doesn't even use the washroom, not once. Obviously a pro. Not me. I'm up and down throughout the flight, excitedly wide awake. I try to sleep but can't. I give up, eating whatever the attendants bring by, and switch on the movie *The Favourite,* impressed as ever with the marvelous Olivia Colman. The plane flies straight toward sunrise, landing in a gray London dawn, iron-colored clouds heaped across an iron-colored sky. Rain pelts the plane as we taxi toward the docking gates.

Shattered with sleeplessness, I make my way to Paddington Station, then my modest hotel that sits kitty-corner to the IASP's conference site, dumping my suitcase on the narrow cot in the cramped room. Fortified with a strong cup of tea, I head outside to explore.

The weather is violently undecided. I walk through a downpour, then sunshine that settles into a soft sideways rain. I look for rainbows but see only pot-bellied storm clouds rolling in, the now slanting rain hitting my face like fine gravel thrown by a malicious hand. It is horrible weather, and thrilling. I am thrilled to be in London.

I wish Simon were with me, but it's an abstract, untruthful wish because part of the thrilling pleasure is in being alone, able to head out into the streets at a moment's notice in terrible weather without making accommodations for a cumbersome wheelchair. I return to the hotel room and drink another steaming cup of tea in silence. Not a single cry of suffering interrupts my caffeinated meditation. I miss Simon, but I don't miss the pain.

I AM STILL THRILLED the following morning as I sit in the conference center listening to Nanna Brix Finnerup, a Danish scientist and chair of the Neuropathic Pain Special Interest Group, deliver the conference's opening remarks to the assembled brain trust of researchers who have arrived from all over the world. She is followed by Lesley Colvin, a pain specialist and professor at the University of Edinburgh, who delivers the morning's first keynote speech, addressing the topic of chemotherapy-induced chronic pain. She begins by relating a story of a patient who survived their cancer but wishes they hadn't because the pain that remained after the chemotherapy systematically destroyed every aspect of their life: one small step forward for cancer treatment that led to two distressing steps backward for patient care and quality of life.

I'm surprisingly moved, sitting in this cavernous ballroom, surrounded by the bespectacled international consortium of clinicians and researchers whose work is to tackle the "global burden of pain." The presentation titles, like the research papers, are often hideously long or sabotaged by a clunky predilection for alliteration, and the language spoken is one I often barely recognize as English. ("Glu-642," one presenter tells us, "is a putative catalytic residue in the active site of the SARM1-TIR enzyme." Sure.)

It would take many years, and a few specialized chemistry degrees, to truly understand the work being shared here. But I'm strangely happy to be among people dedicating their time to understanding pain; happy to be in an environment where pain exists as an objective idea, a problem that can and will be solved; happy in my anonymity to pass, for a few days, as one of the potential solvers of the pain problem instead of one among the voiceless multitude whose lives are affected by real, manifest suffering.

The International Association for the Study of Pain has worked diligently to have chronic pain more officially recognized as a disease state. The World Health Organization, as part of its mandate to advance global health, maintains a compendium of diagnostic codes known as the International Classification of Diseases, or ICD. Since its inception, the ICD has been in a continual state of revision reflecting scientific advances, but neither the present version (ICD-10) nor any previous version has included a systematic representation of chronic pain diagnoses.

For the past six years, an IASP working group has been developing a comprehensive classification for chronic pain, a complex taxonomy that accounts not only for the intensity of pain but also for the compounding factors of pain-related disability, distress, and interference with daily functioning. Several subcommittees, or Special Interest Groups, have helped to refine the proposed definition, creating, for example, various classifications for distinct types of pain: cancer-related, diabetes-related, neuropathic, headache/orofacial, musculoskeletal, or post-surgical. Nanna Brix Finnerup, as head of the Neuropathic Pain Special Interest Group, has played a key role in shaping this new definition, which the IASP has recently submitted to the WHO. The group will learn later this month whether the definition will be included in the upcoming ICD-11.

I meet Dr. Brix Finnerup during the mid-morning break. We've communicated a few times in the weeks before the conference, and the tone of her emails matches her in person: smart, kind, welcoming. Even though she is at the very center of this international gathering and is constantly being diverted by conference-goers wanting to connect, she gives me her focused attention long enough to answer questions about what it will mean to her, as a pain researcher, if the WHO accepts these new definitions.

"Well, there will be a more uniform understanding," she says. "Pain researchers around the world will be using the same classification, which is helpful in collaborations. And we can teach students about pain using this system.

Typically, at medical schools, pain is a neglected area. I hope this change will eventually lead to more and more systematic teachings."

"Why," I ask, "do you think pain is such a neglected area in medical training?"

"Well, generally, pain is only mentioned as a by-product of another specific health issue that is being studied. It is reduced to one of many symptoms and rarely viewed as an issue in its own right."

I ask what it will mean for patients, and how long it will take for the new revisions to affect health policies in various countries. It will take a while, she tells me. Some countries, like the U.S., are still discussing implementing certain revisions made to the ICD-9. But there should be some immediate, specific benefits. For example, when a physician gives a diagnosis of diabetes, other relevant diagnoses that are common in this patient population will pop up on their computer screen for consideration—say, kidney and eye diseases, but also now, painful diabetic neuropathy. Similarly, in an oncology department, after a diagnosis of cancer, painful chemotherapy-induced neuropathy will now be included in the list of potential comorbid conditions a patient might have to deal with. "I hope," Dr. Brix Finnerup says, "that this will raise awareness and make physicians ask more about pain, which in turn will lead to more focus, more understanding, and more requests for education on the topic."

There is much more to discuss, but the coffee break is over. Dr. Brix Finnerup smiles and says she would be happy to talk again. I thank her and head off to my next verbosely titled presentation: "Increasing the Efficiency and Value of Pre-Clinical and Clinical Pain Research to Enhance the Development of Novel Analgesic Therapies for Neuropathic Pain."

BACK IN QUEBEC, Simon's dashed spirits rally. After the crazy post-ablation pain and the disruption of traveling, his TACKLING PAIN routines faltered, but now he writes to tell me he is recommitting to the iom2 meditations and Dreampad time. But, he says, he won't do his regular journaling. Instead he'll send a daily email to me.

> *Kara, my sweet. I miss you. How was your day? Anything interesting happen? I've been reading through the Explain Pain books and it got me thinking . . . I have a question you might want to toss out to all the big brains at the conference: Has there ever been a study looking at the correlation between anxiety-causing news and a spike in chronic pain? Is the demise of our earthly environment and democratic process informing a chronic pain response? Are our molecules sending out an insistent alarm urging us to be more bio-friendly? Is Trump making my back hurt?*
> *—Smooches, Si.*

Later that night, at the networking cocktail reception, waiters glide by with trays of generously filled wineglasses and buttery prawns. Outside, it's still stormy, and I take a few moments to wipe the raindrops off my glasses with the dry edge of a shirtsleeve before grabbing a glass of wine and entering the fray. Around me, people greet one another enthusiastically, friends, colleagues, and collaborators who likely only get to meet in person like this every year or two. As a global consortium of pain experts, the gathered group is relatively small.

I walk around the perimeter of the party, suddenly conscious of my outsider status. I am a scout from the other side—the patient and family side of the pain equation. I'm not here just to socialize or network; what I really want is insider info to take home to Simon. After making a full circuit, I see Julian Taylor, a spinal cord researcher whom Nanna Brix Finnerup introduced me to earlier. I attended his presentation—the only one at the conference specific to spinal cord injury—this afternoon. He presented with Ruth Defrin, a researcher from Israel whose work focused on understanding the underlying physiological mechanism in central neuropathic pain for people with spinal cord injuries. Although the idea that spinal cord injury disrupts the process responsible for both amplifying and reducing the danger signals that modulate the pain response is familiar to Simon, me, and the research world at large, the *how* and *why* of it are still much less clear. Dr. Defrin's research is providing evidence to support the theory that damage to the anterolateral spinothalamic tract is the key precursor to developing central neuropathic pain.

The spinothalamic tract is one of the most important sensory pathways of the nervous system, responsible for transmitting nociceptive, temperature, and crude touch signals; it relays messages to the thalamus, the oval-shaped mass of gray matter deep in the center of the brain. Damage to this critical pathway can amplify hyperexcitable, hyperresponsive danger signals as well as decrease or totally eliminate the inhibitory signals that could reduce pain—a toxic combination that leads to the kind of spontaneous painstorms that Simon so routinely experiences.

Dr. Taylor presented research about the therapeutic use of oleic acid (found in olive oil) in combination with albumin (a type of protein) to prevent pain. The initial results had been promising but were a long way away from having commercial potential.

I reintroduce myself and compliment him on the presentation. He is charming and easy to talk to despite having a bad cold. As the research director at the National Spinal Injuries Centre in the U.K., he is knowledgeable about paralysis, and he asks a few questions about the specifics of Simon's injury. I, in turn, ask what drew him into the field of pain research.

"Fortuitous circumstance, I suppose. As a kid, I thought I would be a veterinarian," he says. "But research opportunities presented themselves..." He shrugs. "I kind of fell into it. Followed the opportunities as they arose. I've been lucky. It's fascinating work."

"Are you aware of any research projects that use virtual reality technology to simulate walking for people who are para- or tetraplegics?" I ask, explaining my brainstorm on the eve of Simon's ablation procedure. "Simon and I were wondering if regular VR exercise might convince his nervous system that he was up and moving again, and that that, in turn, might dampen the pain." Dr. Taylor shakes his head, no. He hasn't heard of any such research. He doesn't seem to think the idea is outrageously far-fetched, though. Or, if he does, he's too polite to say. We return to the topic of his presentation and I ask if he has any idea when something might be made commercially available.

He shakes his head again. "Sadly, no. It's a frustratingly long process."

"Is there something that Simon could take that would mimic the effects in the meantime?" I ask.

"DHA," he says, blowing his nose with admirable delicacy into a tiny cocktail napkin. "You can pick it up at a health food store."

I nod. I'm familiar with DHA—or docosahexaenoic acid—one of the omega-3 fatty acids found in fish oil. It seems an unnecessary bummer to end a pleasant conversation by explaining that Simon has been taking DHA supplements for ten years now, since the time he was in rehab.

I have a brief exchange with a friendly physiotherapist from Australia, and then a man named Willard introduces himself as we both help ourselves to more hors d'oeuvres. Willard is a doctor from Syracuse, New York, who runs a pain management clinic. His energy is intense and his disgust with his patients palpable.

"All of them are fat," he says, stabbing at his helpless prawn with a toothpick. "All of them are hooked on painkillers. I tell them they need to lose thirty pounds and get off the narcotics if they want to get better. But what can you do? They're like children! They don't listen." He swallows a second prawn, then abruptly invites me out for dinner. "Completely innocent, of course," he adds.

Of course. "Thank you, but no," I say, eager to put some space between myself and this terrifically unpleasant person.

AT HOME, HEADLINES, radio shows, and TV news spots have been dominated for some time by the story of what is commonly referred to as the "opioid crisis." Here at the conference I see evidence of my own cultural bias, because apparently within the global community the more accurate term is "the North American opioid crisis."

In 2019, 62 million people, or 1.2 percent of the global population, used opioids for nonmedical purposes. But in North America, that figure is 3.6 percent of the population, the highest rate in the world. At 0.8 percent, Europe has the lowest rate. The geographical disparity also exists in legitimate medical use for opioids—say, in acute care, or post-surgery, or for the palliative treatment of cancer patients or others who face an agonizing death. In 2019, medical professionals in West and Central Africa had access each day to four standard doses of controlled pain medications per million people in their countries, whereas their medical counterparts in North America had access to 36,000 doses per million people each day. Generally, in low- and middle-income countries, doctors are able to access less than 1 percent of the amount of controlled pain medications available in high-income countries, even though lower- and middle-income countries account for 84 percent of the world's population.

The U.S., with just over 4 percent of the world's population, is responsible for roughly 99 percent of global hydrocodone use and 83 percent of oxycodone. The next-highest prescriber of opioids in the world is Canada, where we account for a paltry 0.48 percent of the global population. It can't be argued that the citizens of either the U.S. or Canada experience more pain than citizens of other countries, but it seems we North Americans are unique in our supersized appetite for these pain-numbing drugs.

*Here at the conference there are many questions,* I write in a return email to Simon. *But not a lot of answers and certainly no easy ones. Just as it is for you and me. Despite all the brilliant conversations about epigenetic expressions and Na channels and axonal degeneration and macrophage inflammation, the three key interventions that researchers find effective in treating pain remain the same: mindfulness, movement, and morphine. And morphine, for various reasons, can be problematic. It seems I'm spending a lot of money to be reminded of something we already knew.*

His reply is almost instantaneous: *Really? That's it? Movement and mindfulness is the best they've got?*

AFTER THE CONFERENCE, Simon's cousin Lia arrives from New York. She's a historian finishing up a book that requires her to visit some of England's oldest library collections. When she heard I was going to be in London, she insisted we plan a road trip, a kind of research-vacation. Initially I futzed over the decision to extend my stay. It was a long time to be away. Expensive, too.

"It's true that a vacation doesn't exactly fall within exploring different strategies for tackling pain," she had said to me over the phone. "But maybe—as Si's primary support person—it's not a bad idea for you to take a break?"

Did I need a break? Likely. But after so long in pain-emergency mode, it was hard to imagine the possibility. I realized that my resistance to extending the trip had nothing to do with time or money. "I guess I feel guilty about the prospect of having pain-free fun without Si," I said.

"I know. But you need to get over that."

She was right, of course.

After the conference, we spend a few days seeing the sights in London. We take a boat ride along the Thames, walk the airy spaces of the Tate Modern, and visit the Globe, the third iteration of the theater first built in 1599 by the Lord Chamberlain's Men, the company that Shakespeare wrote for. Still, the problem of pain is ever present in my thoughts, and on our second day of sightseeing, I convince

Lia to visit the Old Operating Theatre Museum and Herb Garret.

St. Thomas' Hospital was built in the twelfth century. The operating theater was established in 1822 in the attic of what was once the hospital's church, and it's the only surviving nineteenth-century operating room in all of Europe. We sit in a cramped horseshoe-shaped gallery looking down on the wooden room where surgeries took place, just as medical students in the 1800s would have done. Museum staff regale us with stories of pre-anesthetic surgeries. Operations, we're told, had to be done quickly before the patient died of blood loss or shock, and a standard post-op treatment might have included "beer, stronger beer, and wine."

The small slant-roofed museum adjacent to the operating theater once housed the herb garret, where medicinal remedies were prepared, such as the one used by royal physician Richard Mead to treat syphilis ("Garden Snails cleansed and bruised, 6 gallons, and Earthworms washed and bruised, 3 gallons"). Although evidence of poppies—the source of opium—was found in this herbal apothecary, along with lavender, peppermint, cloves, and a variety of other plants, opium (or any of its derivatives) was not routinely used until the tail end of the nineteenth century. Before that, surgery, with no real pain-relieving option available, was a horror. Novelist Fanny Burney provides a detailed account of this horror in a letter written to her sister describing the successful mastectomy she underwent in 1810, with nothing stronger than a glass of wine cordial to mitigate the pain of amputation.

The doctors, Fanny explained in the letter, had cautioned her not to attempt to withhold her screams. "Yet—when the dreadful steel was plunged into the breast—cutting though veins—arteries—flesh—nerves—I needed no injunctions not to restrain my cries. I began a scream that lasted unintermittingly during the whole time of the incision—& I almost marvel that it rings not in my Ears still! so excruciating was the agony," Fanny wrote. "When the wound was made, & the instrument was withdrawn, the pain seemed undiminished, for the air that suddenly rushed into those delicate parts felt like a mass of minute but sharp and forked poniards, that were tearing the edges of the wound." The doctors, she states, were forced to cut against the grain of the breast tissue, the flesh so insistently resisting the knife that the surgeon quickly tired and was forced to alternately use his left and right hands. Several times, Fanny concluded that the "speechless torture" of the surgery must be over, only to have the surgeon, after a brief rest, renew his efforts, until finally she experienced the disordering sensation of the "knife rackling against the bone—scraping it!"

"Can you imagine?" I ask Lia, as we climb down the steep spiral staircase back to the busy London streets. "An anesthetic-less mastectomy?"

"Nope," she says. "And I don't want to try."

OUR ROAD TRIP takes us as far north as Edinburgh, and then we circle back to Penrith, a small city on the northern border of the Lake District where Lia lived for several years. We're stopping to visit an old friend of hers, John Alderson, who has graciously agreed to talk to me about his experience of pain in the aftermath of a cancer diagnosis. Like the patient profiled in the opening remarks of the Neuropathic Pain conference, John responded well to his treatment protocol, making an unexpected recovery from his cancer, but it's a recovery that has come at a very high cost.

John worked as a postman, raising a family with his wife, Val, in the small community where Lia and her husband, Edmund, lived. The four became fast friends, and Lia adored John for his gregarious personality. He was a natural storyteller, the guy in the room who made people laugh and feel at ease. "Personality-wise, he's a lot like Simon," Lia says now as we reach the outskirts of Penrith. "Life of the party."

In 2006 a malignant tumor was discovered on the left side of John's neck, and then a second one buried under his clavicle. Treatment was aggressive: surgery, radiotherapy, and chemotherapy. At the time, it was unclear what to expect. "We thought, at best, it was going to buy him more time," Lia explains. But, amazingly, the cancer didn't return. And when he didn't die he became an interesting case study in what, exactly, were the long-term effects of his intense radiotherapy treatment.

These effects, it turned out, were catastrophic. The surgery resulted in extensive nerve damage to his left shoulder and arm, and the radiotherapy resulted in excruciating neck pain. His doctor apologized for instantly giving John the neck of someone twice his age. John's throat also closed, limiting his ability to swallow, and he was fitted with a feeding tube. Over the next few years, he experimented with eating small amounts of soup and liquids along with the nutritional guck that was pumped through the tube. But even ingesting the smallest amount of real food resulted in particles being aspirated into his lungs, which in turn resulted in increasingly more dangerous forms of pneumonia. Then his trachea began to spasm, making proper inhalation and exhalation impossible. A tracheostomy was performed, a tube placed in his throat to better help him breathe.

Lia has prepared me with this backstory but still, when we arrive, John's level of disability is shocking. He is hooked to an oxygen machine by a long tube, a kind of oversized umbilical cord that snakes through the rooms of his home, allowing him to move about. He needs to plug the trach to issue his greeting, and I can see the effort required to speak out loud is tremendous. Still, he is warm and welcoming, a cheekiness in his grin as he gives Lia a bear hug. He asks about Simon, wondering how he's managing while I'm away.

"I've never met him," John says. "But, after talking with Lia, I feel a certain connection."

John has been making his negotiations with the beast of pain for thirteen years. Initially, when he came out of the hospital, he was prescribed extremely high doses of morphine. After a few years, as he slowly recovered from the ravages of surgery, chemo, and radiation and—unexpectedly—didn't die, he became more aware of the high he experienced with the morphine and began to crave it all the time. Then he did something he never would have believed possible: he began to sneak extra doses, adding water to the morphine bottle like a teenager diluting his parents' vodka. His wife, Val, caught on and confronted him. He was mortified, and together they agreed it was best if she alone was responsible for such a powerful drug. She stored it in a locked cabinet and adhered to administering it on a strict schedule.

Over the years there have been ebbs and flows in John's nerve pain, which he describes as feeling like nettle stings times a thousand. Like Simon and me, he and Val have felt isolated in their rural community, and it was difficult and time-consuming to connect with medical practitioners who specialized in treating neuropathic pain. Things reached a crisis point when he and Val relocated and his new doctor abruptly stopped his morphine prescription. The pain raged and John was incapacitated for weeks. Val rang his doctor, who consistently refused to visit, repeatedly stating that John's pain was not real but brought on by his extreme situation. "She told me the pain was all in my head. She thought I was craving opioids," John says. "But all I was craving was pain relief, in whatever form."

Something had to be done, and thankfully they found a new doctor, one who helped gradually wean John from the morphine, replacing it with tramadol and gabapentin, one of the few drugs that is effective in treating nerve pain.

We talk a little about the ways in which his pain is intimately connected to a worry that the cancer will return and the losses he has experienced. Initially John thought the feeding tube was a temporary measure, and it didn't bother him. But reckoning with its permanence was much more difficult.

"Being told I wouldn't eat again was not easy to get my head around, and the truth is I haven't and never will. I still crave food every day," he explains in a whisper. "Food is all around us: advertising, books, cooking programs. Family celebrations. Christmastime is weird."

It's hard to imagine. Simon is no stranger to permanent injuries, to living a life where "all better" isn't an option, yet when I think of how much both he and I rely on the daily routines of planning, preparing, and enjoying a meal together to structure and bring pleasure to difficult days—it's a loss that seems inconceivable.

And yet, looking at John's smiling face, apparently not. When I ask what gets him through his days, his list is long and varied. Like Simon, he loves watching sports. And like Simon, he is a musician, and though he's unable to play because of the nerve damage in his left arm, listening provides endless pleasure. He's revisited the poetry he studied in school and finds himself powerfully moved in new and unexpected ways. Though he can't eat, he enjoys cooking for Val. And he loves documentaries, especially anything to do with Alaska and Canada. We spend a good while comparing notes on our favorite Netflix series. Like us, he and Val have found good therapeutic benefit in various BBC crime dramas.

"Without a doubt, though," he whispers, "the main factor in me managing my situation is how amazing Val is. I could go on forever and a day about her. I'm sure Simon would agree: it's a big deal to know you always have someone *there* for you. And my kids, Becky and Neil. They are a massive part of what keeps me going. They are grown now and living life to the full. They have good jobs and things they love to do. That they are happy means everything. It helps me handle the moments of depression and pain. If they were struggling, I don't know exactly how that would impact me, but I know it would."

John explains that he and Val have turned into professional form-filler-inners. But, he tells me, it's a small price to pay for the blessing of the National Health Service. The services provided by the NHS, along with the pension he receives from the Royal Mail, mean that while he and Val are not wealthy, they are okay.

"If you have a comfortable home," he says, "that goes a long way in helping you cope with things you previously could never have imagined."

He's tired now, and Lia gives me a pointed look: it's time for us to leave. John thanks me as we say our goodbyes. "The impact of my health problems on all our lives has been immense. It's hard to convey, isn't it?" he says. "To people who aren't in a similar situation. When you do it can sound like you're moaning, but—facts are facts. It feels good to talk about it."

"It's me who should be thanking you," I say.

John nods, his voice exhausted, then manages to add: "You can email any time."

"I never know when I see John," Lia says, as we pull away, "if it will be the last time. These visits have become incredibly precious."

We both fall silent to our own internal thoughts as she weaves through the narrow Penrith streets. It strikes me that Simon and John are similar in ways beyond their outgoing personalities. Even after a brief conversation, it's evident that John, like Simon, worries more about his wife and children than he does about himself. It's a remarkable thing: to be in such extreme pain and yet not privilege it over the potential pain of others. For a wild moment, I imagine this mindset as a kind of river underneath the river of their lives, a subterranean current of grace that has helped them flow through unimaginable difficulties. It is a lesson for me, and one I hope I remember if—when—I am in a situation of enduring great pain.

"There's a strength that Simon and John share," I say to Lia, breaking our silence.

She nods, momentarily preoccupied with finding the turnoff that will return us to the highway. We're on our way to Heathrow, where she'll take a return flight to New York and I'll hop another red-eye for a brief layover in Quebec before Simon and I head back home.

"Valiant," she says, merging into the southbound traffic. "*Valiant* is the word that comes to mind."

# 14

# Time Is Art

MAY 25, DAY 307.

Today the World Health Organization officially adopts the latest revision of the International Classification of Diseases, the ICD-11, which now includes a comprehensive definition of chronic pain as a disease.

Around the world, and throughout history, countless people have visited their physicians in agony, only to be told—because there was no official code to diagnose it or clear way to objectively measure it—that somehow their pain was less than real. There is power in being able to name something, especially if that something is immense, invisible, and threatening.

At dinner, over homemade mushroom-and-rosemary pizzas, we toast the ICD-11, then I read out loud one of Simon's recent journal entries that intrigued me:

> *It's taking a while for me to fully absorb the difficult fact that if the brain is the theater master in the house of pain, then I am always both the cure and the disease. Given the nature of some of the strategies we've been dabbling in, it seems that bearing witness to chronic pain has the potential to be both helpful* AND *harmful.*

"Helpful *and* harmful?" I say. "How so?"

"Well, this past year has helped me, I know," he says. "It's not really measurable or quantifiable, but things are better. Having concrete things to do, like the iom2 meditations, makes me feel as if I have a small amount of agency within an experience that still falls largely out of my control. But..." he pauses, shading his eyes. We're eating out on the porch, evening sun slanting directly into his face. Across the street a baby is crying. "It's harmful in that you never want to give pain *too* much airtime. I don't want it to be the only thing we talk or think about. Also, sometimes just thinking or talking about pain seems to set it off. Aggressive redirection is valuable, I think. Really, I'd like to never say that word—*pain*—again. Just remove it from my vocabulary."

"No kidding," I say. "The idea that you're the cure *and* the disease is interesting too."

Simon laughs. "I'll tell you what: I thought three things in quick succession after I wrote that. First, I thought, wow, this journaling thing is working. I really figured out something *true* here. I really *nailed* it. Then I thought, I can't wait to show this to Kara because it makes me sound super-smart and all pain-philosophical. Then, last thought, I realized it was totally dumb and not right or true at all."

"Okay," I say. "Explain."

"Well, neither word—*cure* or *disease*—is right. How can you *cure* pain? It is an essential part of being alive. It's not even possible. *Disease* is a little trickier. I can see how important it is from a clinical point of view to have that clarification of chronic pain as a disease for the ICD," Simon says. "But recently I've been thinking how important it is for me *not* to think of pain as a disease. Or, at least, to think of it as something separate from my spinal cord injury. I mean, I have to live with this bum back. The wheelchair. It took a while to be reconciled with that. But maybe the pain is different."

"Maybe you don't have to accept it?" I say.

"Well. I don't know about that. The pain is what it is. I need to keep trying to move through it. Try to make it better, not worse."

"That is... wise."

"Ha! You don't have to sound so surprised," Simon says. "The thing is, thinking about my pain as a disease makes me worry that I suffer a little from Stockholm syndrome, that in some insidious way I'll become attached to its permanence. I don't want to be. I don't have to be. Neither of us does. Even if it persists. Does that make sense?"

"Sure," I say. "But that's a tough place to be in."

"I guess. But the pain started suddenly. And, for myself, the biggest takeaway from the past year is that I need to work hard to keep open the possibility that it might also stop suddenly. Why not? It's unlikely, maybe, but not impossible." A flurry of unspoken thoughts passes across his face like sudden storm clouds.

"What?" I say. "What is it?"

"Well," he says. "It's just, you're right. It's a tough place to be in. I'm so glad we undertook this experiment. It's helped, you know, feeling more connected with you in confronting the pain. And I know you've put in hours of research and time with me, so I'm not complaining. But the reality is that dealing with my stupid body takes up all of my time. Every day, my morning routine can take anywhere from three to five hours, more if my unpredictable bowels decide to surprise me. Then the pain interventions take up another big chunk of time. If I teach a guitar lesson, or two, that's it, that's my day. It's time to start making dinner and thinking about bedtime. It's such an extraordinary amount of work for such a small result."

"I'm so sorry, Beau," I say. "It sucks."

"Yep," he nods. "Pain sucks. Every minute of every day."

"It's the title of your autobiography: *Pain Sucks: Every Minute of Every Day.*"

"Truth, baby," Simon says.

"Partly the pain intervention stuff takes up so much time because it's new and we're struggling to figure it out. The more you do it, the more consistent you can be, the easier it will get. Ideally all the neuroplastic techniques will start to integrate into your daily routine, easy as flossing your teeth."

"Fuck," Si says. "I should do that more too."

"Did you talk to Dr. Jaschinski today?" I ask, working hard to keep my tone neutral. I don't want to sound too eager, or anxious. It's time to renew his hydromorphone prescription, but Simon has been waffling. Over the past ten months we've continued to discuss the possibility that his opioid prescription might be doing as much to maintain his pain levels as to ameliorate them. Would the neuroplastic techniques or the mindfulness practices be more effective if Simon were opioid-free? I want to give it a try. Simon is less enthusiastic.

"Yep," he says, his tone glum. "I didn't request a higher dose, even though I could use one. Instead we talked about safe ways of weaning myself off. He suggested lowering the dose slowly, in two-milligram increments. I'm going to give it a shot, but no promises. We'll see how it goes."

"Agreed," I say. "You know, we're coming up to a full year of our pain project. What do you think? Do we keep going?"

"Oh baby, that's cute," Si says. "Do we have a choice?"

I'M RELIEVED THAT Simon is still committed to our project. While I was traveling, my own journal entries kept returning to a troubling question that eerily echoed Simon's own insights. Was my expectation of—my insistence on—continued healing something that helped Simon? Or harmed him? When he was weary with pain, was the hope I held on his behalf a gift, or just another burden? Inside the contradictory world of chronic pain, I am starting to see it is always a bit of both.

I reach out to Lorimer Moseley in his hometown of Sydney, Australia. Along with David Butler, Professor Moseley is responsible for the comprehensive research in the Explain Pain series that has provided the scaffold for the self-propelled educational upgrade Simon and I have undergone. The books are dense but engaging—an incredible resource for a person-in-pain, or a loved one of a person-in-pain, or a health care provider. They don't leave many questions unanswered, but there are two key things I want to ask.

The Explain Pain series resisted calling chronic pain a disease, a position I found refreshing. And I'm wondering, in Professor Moseley's opinion, is the IASP's expanded definition of chronic pain as a disease, and its subsequent acceptance into the ICD-11, a good thing?

"I think yes," he says, responding by email. He cites the ways in which the expanded definition might open funding to provide high-value care, but he cautions that it's not an entirely risk-free development. "Any opportunity for improving services and care for people in pain often comes with an opportunity for making money from *appearing* to provide such services and care. That is, I reckon we can see a shift in marketing approaches by, say, the neurostimulation device makers, and indeed other drug makers—Lyrica, for example—to position themselves as an alternative to opioids. But the evidence is not nearly as helpful as they claim."

Purdue Pharma launched a new era of medical marketing with its aggressive strategy to promote the painkiller OxyContin. Professor Moseley describes how current promotional campaigns use similar tactics—mass media blitzes, doctor lunches, and perks—noting that device companies are not bound by the same regulation as the pharmaceutical industry. "So, I think the expanding definition has a risk of opening a door for commercially driven, cashed-up players to push it wider," he says. "The sad reality is that if we provide the care we are meant to—with a focus on understanding, empowerment, enablement, activity, and self-management—no one really makes money."

The second question I ask is more personal. The introduction to *Explain Pain* states that the "principles presented in this book are particularly suited to consideration of chronic non-specific pain (e.g. low back pain, elbow pain)." I'm certain *Explain Pain* would have helped me during my decade-long experience with low back and sciatica pain. And I think the knowledge I've gained in its pages will help me face whatever pain awaits me in the future, whether acute or chronic.

But how applicable is an *Explain Pain* educational program for someone like Simon? In engaging in this ongoing pain experiment, have we been setting him up for yet one more colossally failed intervention? I explain to Professor Moseley how Simon suffered the hat trick of central nervous system injury, with damage done to the brain, the brain stem, and the spinal cord. Does it make a difference, I ask, if the original insult is to the nervous system itself?

"I think it does make a difference," he says. "However, this is notoriously difficult. But the principles should be the same. I would think continued peppering of Simon's nervous system to convince it that there is no benefit to protective behavior should slowly help. I wonder about things like going hard on exercise, but I am completely naive to Simon, of course. It's a very, very tricky situation that you both must find frustrating. I can only say—patience, persistence, and courage—even injured nervous systems can change."

It's a thoughtful response, and a validating one. It helps.

SIMON AND I AGREE our next step is to set up some exercise routines, but he is, to say the least, resistant to moving ahead with this next phase of our TACKLING PAIN plan. It's tough. We've been together for almost thirty years, and though we are very different people, we normally exist in an easygoing, mutually aligned state. But on this issue our perspectives are worlds apart. I grew up in dance studios, a lifelong student of various movement practices. Simon, on the other hand, would prefer to undergo a root canal than take an exercise class. I have on occasion considered pushing him, as Lorimer Moseley suggested, to go hard on exercising, but I also haven't wanted to be *that* person in his life—and everyone knows at least one of them—the smug asshole who tells the chronically ill person that they'd feel better if only they exercised more.

The science is clear: exercise is good for you. We all know this. *Motion,* as almost every handbook on chronic pain will tell you, *is lotion*. Regular movement promotes resiliency in both muscle and connective tissue. It promotes circulation of both blood and lymphatic fluids, which in turn boosts the body's healing and immune processes. Mental health, heart health, joint health, muscle strength, bone density, posture, and proprioceptive awareness all benefit from regular movement. But it's also true that a suitable exercise program for someone with chronic pain may not be easily accessible. And for someone navigating the multiple demands of an injured and/or ill body, exercising may feel neither meaningful nor compelling.

Simon's never liked the concept of exercise. That isn't to say that, before his accident, he wasn't fit. He was. He had a natural kinetic sense and a strong physical presence as a performing musician. He maintained his health by being active in his life: working in construction, parenting an athletic kid, playing music. But he was never inclined to play competitive sports, and the idea of booking time to go to the gym to "work out" was, for him, ridiculous. And now the thought of exercise—after brain and spinal cord injury—is that much more unappealing.

"Look," he says now. "I know this is something I have to do. But that's just it. It's one more thing I *have* to do to take care of this stupid body."

"Is that all?"

"What do you mean?"

"Well, I've been thinking about what you said before—that the prospect of facing your physical limitations made you sad, which then made you mad, and you hated feeling sad-mad. The same is true for me. I should be supporting you more, pushing you even, with exercise. But I don't because, one, I don't want to nag. But, if I'm honest, even more than that, it also makes me sad-mad. I don't like how tough it is for you. I guess, most of the time, I'd like to ignore that reality."

Simon nods.

"I miss your old body," I say.

"Oh, Stan," Si says, grabbing my hands. "I miss it too."

"I'm not going to cry."

"Me either."

"Okay, then. Let's think more *movement practice* and less *exercise regime.*"

"And the difference is...?"

"Well, a movement practice is about calming and re-energizing the nervous system through intentional awareness and movement education. Whereas in an exercise regime, you impose your will on yourself to do enough crunches and squats that you'll look good hitting the beach."

"Okay. My vanity days are over. Movement practice it is. Where should we start?"

"Simple," I say. "Super simple. Remember what Les Aria said about not being able to teach in a storm? That's where we start: gentle movement that can ease you through the storm. Because we know, for sure, there will be a bit of a storm when you first start moving."

"Okay. Let's try swimming," he says.

Our small swim-spa has been turned off all winter, but now I clean the cover, turn up the heat, and test the pH balance. In the past, the gravity-friendly environment of the water has provided good movement opportunities for Simon, but last summer even that was too much for him. The difficult transfer of paralyzed limbs in and out of the tub, the hot water jets hitting his back, the unfolding of his body from his usual seated posture—all these things triggered massive waves of pain.

So this time we start more slowly. For the first few days, I assist him in the transfer into the tub and then support him as he floats. He doesn't attempt to swim, or stretch, but instead focuses on a breathing exercise, inhaling to a count of four and then slowly exhaling on a count of twelve. It is a deep diaphragmatic breath that is, on a physiological level, a readily available and risk-free antidote to stress.

This increase in activity alone causes an initial spike in pain, but after two weeks of committing to a regular schedule, it evens out. By week three, he is able to transfer independently and adds five minutes of swimming. The next week, he's up to ten. It's a good start.

"I'm getting through the storm," he says.

"How is it feeling? I ask. "Like a chore? Or are you having fun?"

"'Fun' is a strong word," he says, smiling. "But, yeah. It's good."

"That should be our goal, right?" I say. "That's it's mostly fun. And that it makes you feel stronger. Joseph Pilates called it the 'return to life.' Exercise should be something that supports you in doing the things you actually want to do, namely play guitar with reduced pain."

"You know what would be fun *and* empowering? If I had a robotic exoskeleton and I could stomp around the garden, or play a gig, like a musical Iron Man. I'm pretty sure if I was up and ambulating, a lot of my pain would disappear."

"Agreed." Unfortunately, robotic exoskeletons, while increasingly becoming viable, aren't an option yet. Maybe in the future. In the meantime, I've still been thinking about how virtual reality technology could help Simon, and I search online for any academic articles about its therapeutic use. Several describe various interventions for both acute and chronic pain, usually implementing either mindfulness meditation or a problem-solving approach in the VR environment. So far, the data is inconclusive but tends to support the theory that VR interventions are more immediately helpful for acute pain.

I find only one paper specific to VR interventions for people with spinal cord injuries. It describes a preclinical experiment, reminiscent of Ramachandran's mirror box, that uses a visual illusion to create a sense of embodiment in paralyzed limbs. The key contact for the study is neuroscientist Olaf Blanke, who is the Bertarelli Foundation Chair in Cognitive Neuroprosthetics at the École Polytechnique Fédérale de Lausanne. Dr. Blanke responds quickly to my email and agrees to chat over Zoom.

When we digitally connect a week later, Dr. Blanke's explanation of the illusion created in the experiment is not difficult to understand. In fact, it's elegant in its simplicity. Participants sit in their wheelchair wearing a head-mounted display and headphones. Fake legs are placed in another wheelchair equipped with a mounted camera, presenting an image that corresponds to the participant's viewpoint, looking down at seated legs.

This image is fed into the head-mounted display so that the dummy legs are superimposed over the participant's physical (paralyzed) legs. An experimenter simultaneously strokes the dummy legs and the participant's back at the lowest level where their normal sensation is preserved. In the VR world, the participant sees their leg being stroked while feeling the tactile stimulation on their back. Although it doesn't persist after the experiment, during the trial participants noted a reduction in neuropathic pain.

"It was encouraging," Dr. Blanke explains. "The tactile stimulation lasted only about a minute, so a very short time. The hope is that with a similar intervention but one of a longer duration, and more routinized—say, fifteen minutes three times a week—the effects might be more pronounced and longer lasting."

It is thrillingly similar to the VR intervention Simon and I imagined so many months ago, only instead of using movement, it uses tactile stimulation. Dr. Blanke listens patiently as I explain the vision we had of paralyzed knees lifting and lowering, or tapping out a dance rhythm, all in a virtual landscape. "What do you think?" I ask. "Is that crazy, far-fetched nonsense?"

He laughs out loud. "No. Not at all. I believe that is the type of direction the technology will move in. We're just not quite there yet."

IT'S DISAPPOINTING THAT an interactive, potentially fun, VR intervention is not yet available. But the positive results of Dr. Blanke's research prompt Simon and me to wonder if we could approximate our hypothetical VR experiment with a form of intense mental exercise. We decide that along with Si's daily meditation, we'll add a regime in which I guide Simon through a series of *imagined* movements. He closes his eyes as I prompt him to mentally go through the motions of flexing and extending his spine and imagining the sensation of the weight of his feet in the footrest, the back of his thighs resting on his wheelchair seat, or the action of raising and lowering a knee.

The benefit of mentally performing an exercise has long been recognized in the dance and movement world.

Feldenkrais practitioners, for example, will often guide a student in imagining a gesture. This practice of mental imagery was extensively explored by a dancer named Mabel Todd, who in 1937 published *The Thinking Body,* a classic text that examined the relationship between cognitive processes and human movement. This evolved into the somatic practice known as ideokinesis (from the Greek *ideo*, meaning "thought," and *kinesis,* meaning "movement"). Long before the term *neuroplasticity* was coined, Mabel (and the teachers she inspired—Lulu Sweigard, Barbara Clark, Irene Dowd, and Eric Franklin, to name a few) recognized that all human body movement is directed by the activity of the nervous system, and that for someone to change ingrained movement patterns, there must first be a change in their thinking. As Irene Dowd writes, "Visualizing a line of movement through the body while *not* moving can change the habitual patterns of messages being sent from the brain through nerve pathways to the muscles."

While the efficacy of an ideokinesis practice has long been intuited by dancers and athletes wanting to improve their physical performance, it was never studied in the kind of broad, rigorous, peer-reviewed way that is required as evidential proof. But the scientific world has started to catch up. In 1995, Alvaro Pascual-Leone, a researcher at Harvard Medical School, published a groundbreaking study demonstrating how the brain changes with the act of simply imagining movement. The study consisted of two groups of people, each being taught the same one-handed sequence of notes on the piano. The first group practiced the sequence for two hours every day for five days; the second group, for the exact same amount of time, only *imagined* playing the sequence. Throughout the five days Pascual-Leone tracked the brain function of both groups using transcranial magnetic stimulation, or TMS, with surprising results: the group that only imagined practicing learned to play the piece almost as well as those who actually practiced, and both groups showed similar changes in brain function. "Mental practice alone seems sufficient to promote the modulation of neural circuits involved in the early stages of motor skill learning," Pascual-Leone writes in the study's summary. "This modulation not only results in marked performance improvement but also seems to place the subjects at an advantage for further skill learning with minimal physical practice."

"See," I say to Simon. "It's all about trying to do more with less effort. Work smarter, as they say, not harder."

Simon nods. "That's an approach to working out that I'm down with."

Two hours of mental practice a day is more than either of us is willing to commit to, and so we aim for a more reasonable fifteen minutes. It's doable, and there are moments when this work of visualizing movement is calming for both of us. But it can also be onerous for me, yet one more thing to squeeze into a busy day, and I struggle with fulfilling my various roles: supportive partner, movement coach, exercise nag. Deciding we need some outside help, Simon books private qigong sessions with a man named Paul Blakey.

Qigong is a centuries-old form of movement meditation, the slow flow of movement and breath designed to cultivate a sense of harmony with nature, both internally (deep inside our individual mysterious bodies) and externally (as we rove the wide, wild world). Paul and Simon practice a series of twelve movements with whimsical names: the Yak, the Waterwheel, the Grand Gesture. Simon has to run through them every day, and he dutifully creates his own calendar, crossing off the days with a large X. Every two or three weeks, Paul comes to check in, encouraging Simon to focus on his breath as a way of rebuilding his energy reserves.

"Making neuroplastic shifts in your pain requires a great deal of energy—or qi—but if that energy isn't there, or is dangerously depleted, well, then it complicates your ability to make any kind of change," Paul says. Initially Simon experiences some uncomfortable surges of excess pain after doing the movement series, but the lyrical gestures are engaging enough that he persists, gradually building his strength and range of motion. But the most delightful thing about the qigong experience, Simon says, is that Paul signs off all his emails with the beautiful phrase *Time Is Art.*

OVER THE COURSE of the following month, Simon has more restful sleeps than usual, and his energy and mood improve dramatically. So do mine.

"I feel as if there's been a huge emotional release for both of us in acknowledging how resistant we were to pushing you to move," I say to Simon, at our next TACKLING PAIN meeting.

He agrees. "I think I had this belief that if exercise wasn't going to give me my old body back, well, then, fuck it. But I feel better. The pain hasn't shifted that much, but something in me has. I'm more like myself."

"Do you have any specific exercise goals going ahead?" I ask.

"My arms are doing double duty as arms *and* legs," Si says. "I guess, aside from reducing overall pain, a key goal is trying to keep my shoulders healthy. Can you help me with that?"

After feeling so powerless for so long in helping Simon address his pain, I'm thrilled with this request. "I can, absolutely," I say.

So, on top of all our other interventions, we add three simple movement patterns meant to release neck and shoulder tension and counteract the daily forces (rolling in the wheelchair, playing guitar, tensing from spikes of pain) that are rounding Simon's shoulders and spine forward. We set a "relaxation alarm" on his Fitbit for every two hours as a cue to take five, or fifteen, minutes to run through these exercises.

It's a lot, really. But Si manages to stick to the every-two-hour schedule, mostly. Next we brainstorm movement options where the fun might outweigh the doing-this-because-it's-good-for-me factor. Simon points out the window at the freestanding basketball net that we bought for Eli on his tenth birthday.

"Hoops?"

"Solid," I say.

I buy a basketball and in the early evenings, before dinner, we play a modified game of twenty-one. Our shot-taking is passable, but Simon has an all-star on-court flex. We gleefully debate the positions where Raptors coach Nick Nurse would slot us in.

"Nick would park you in the offensive end and tell the rest of the team to get you the ball," I say.

"Just call me Wheels McSwish," he says as I grab his rebound, jumping up for my signature move: the skyhook.

"Nice," he says. "You'll be Stanley Buckets."

"Wheels McSwish and Stanley Buckets: I like it. Can we get T-shirts made?"

Occasionally pain spikes disrupt these new activities. But overall Simon is able to stay consistent, and his confidence in his physical body is so bolstered that he jumps at an unexpected opportunity to try out adaptive paddleboarding, something he has rigorously avoided in the past. So this is how we find ourselves, on a sunny afternoon, paddling out into the clear water of the Sechelt Inlet.

We're guided by Jordan Kerton, owner of Access Revolution (a self-described "social-impact business" that specializes in hiking and paddling adventures for people of all abilities), and local paddling guru Geordie Harrower. Simon and I are on a specially designed board wide enough to accommodate his wheelchair and outfitted with two side pontoons for stability. I stand at the front of the board, at first a little nervous. The ocean is unpredictable, and Simon's wheelchair...? Well, it could hardly be called buoyant. But the board is remarkably stable, and after a few clunky moments we manage to coordinate our paddling, gliding though the water easily.

Up ahead an eagle soars out of the shaggy arms of the shoreline cedars, then dives toward the water's crinkled surface, talons reaching to grab a fish.

"He caught his lunch," Simon says.

"How are you doing?" I ask, glancing over my shoulder.

"I'm kind of... exhilarated. I mean, this is where we live," Si says. He gestures with his paddle at the sea, the sky, the forest, and the distant mountains. "It's not too shabby."

# 15

# The Meaning of Pain

MAY 28, DAY 310.

Simon does an over-the-shoulder check as the ferry traffic merges onto the highway. "We're taking the Lonsdale exit, right?"

"Yep," I say, double-checking on Google Maps. We're following Eli's directions to a cannabis dispensary in Vancouver, where we plan to drop a couple of hundred dollars on various edibles. Eli claims that this dispensary is particularly skilled at coming up with unique concoctions for people with complex pain issues. "I think they might be able to help Dad," he said over the phone. "But I don't know how much longer they'll be operating, so my advice is to bring cash, and bring a lot."

Simon is looking for contingencies as he attempts to cut back on his hydromorphone use but is adamant about not wanting to feel high, a sensation that since his head injury he finds deeply unpleasant. Already Dr. Jaschinski has prescribed Sativex, a pharmaceutical spray that combines THC and CBD, the active ingredients in cannabis that help promote pain relief. Simon has found it marginally helpful, but it's difficult to accurately regulate the dose. It's easy, in the spray form, to overdo it; one half-squirt too many and he's unhappily stoned. Eli is certain this store might provide better options. So this is why, on a busy day of responsible, adult errands, we've prioritized finding the dispensary to buy some dope.

It's not illegal, exactly, what we're doing. In fact, Canada just became the second country in the world (Uruguay was the first) to legalize marijuana for not only medical but also recreational use, and the cannabis equivalent to provincially owned liquor stores now exist in most communities across the country. But even before legalization, British Columbia had one of the most pro-pot cultures in the world. "B.C. bud" has an international reputation, and local strains of weed—Texada Timewarp, for example, a hardy outdoor plant—are world-renowned for their potency and pain-killing properties. In fact, B.C.'s robust black-market pot culture has complicated legalization and is part of the reason that storefront cannabis dispensaries like the one Eli has directed us to are operating, at least temporarily, in a legal gray zone.

These stores proliferated across the province in the early 2000s, when British Columbians topped the nation as legit medical-marijuana users. Lining their shelves with glass jars filled with various cannabis strains, these dispensaries were the newest iteration of an alternative apothecary, the skunk-like smell of weed so dense it would cling to your hair and clothes long after you exited the premises. But now, with legalization, cannabis dispensaries need a government license to operate, which is both expensive and hard to obtain. Without licenses, they are operating, technically, on the wrong side of the law. It's easy to imagine that in the near future, these dispensaries will be entirely replaced by the government-sanctioned cannabis stores, but for now, Eli suggests we take advantage of their broader range of products.

The benefits of pot for certain people have been widely recognized and, long before legalization, supported by elaborate compassionate care networks that procured cannabis for the chronically or terminally ill. When we were in our early twenties, Simon worked for a brief time in a hydroponic store. Although it was a legitimate business (selling supplies for indoor greenhouses), it serviced a then illegal but thriving underground pot-growing industry. Simon would return home at night and regale me with the epic claims made by cannabis enthusiasts. "Pot," he told me, "is apparently a one-stop healing shop. It cures everything! Insomnia, anxiety, depression? It'll fix it. Glaucoma, arthritis, epilepsy? Got you covered. High blood pressure, heart disease, a touch of a tumor? No problem. Add a sprinkle of pixie dust, it'll cure your asthma too."

International medical science, so far, does not wholly agree. There is a paucity of peer-reviewed studies on the benefits and risks of cannabis, and the ones that do exist do not offer unqualified recommendations for its therapeutic use. These studies contend that the potential health risks of routine cannabis use, like *increased* depression, anxiety, suicidal ideation, or cancer, have still not been properly investigated. In Canada, doctors can authorize patients to procure cannabis for medical reasons, but they cannot broadly prescribe it in its many forms of ingestion, unless it is, like Sativex, a government-registered medication.

"There's not enough quality data for medical science to get totally on board yet," I told Simon when we began discussing the possibility of adding cannabis to his daily pain-relieving arsenal.

"Well," he said, "I guess we're going to have to figure it out ourselves."

This is a sentiment that has lately peppered our TACKLING PAIN conversations. It's a change in attitude that is helping us make the transition from the question *what is pain?* to *what does this pain mean to us?*

David Morris argues in the seminal book *The Culture of Pain* that the human physical experience of pain is inextricably tied to the cerebral construction of its meaning, a meaning that exists "within the shifting process of human culture and of individual minds." Pain, Morris tells us, "is never simply a sensation but rather something that the time-bound brain interprets and that the time-bound mind constructs: a specific human artifact bearing the mark of its specific human history."

As products of twenty-first-century North American society, Simon and I would describe our primary cultural inheritance as one that views pain as an unacceptable inconvenience. No one—not doctors, not patients, not insurers, not employers—has time for persistent pain, and we, as a society of consumers, believe ourselves to be entitled to (as the endless ads promise) *fast, easy, immediate* relief.

The prescription that Lorimer Moseley suggested in his email—to provide understanding, empowerment, enablement, activity, and self-management—would require a significant cultural shift in public health policy. Healing would take *time,* and it would require greater social investment in providing pain education, broad holistic health resources, job retraining, and flexible work reentry programs.

"Off the top of your head, quick reaction: What would you say pain means to you right now?" I ask Simon as we drive along the highway.

"Vulnerability," he says. "It's the experience of lacking moment-by-moment control over this thing that exerts such a massive influence in my life. What does it mean to you?"

"I guess, right now, it means limits. Limits to your healing from the accident. Limits to what I can do to help you."

"We're not really a society that likes the idea of limits," Si says. "Or vulnerability."

"Right? Limits are due to a lack of ambition. Or a failure of imagination or intellect," I say. "I've bought into that idea more than I realized but... now? It seems childish."

"Yeah," Si says. "Life in a chair has definitely changed my perspective. It's all about figuring out what are the self-imposed limitations you need to challenge and what are the ones you need to find a way to live with. Not all limitations are inherently defeatist. They are just... reasonable."

"And your pain, with its associations of vulnerability and limitations, is so different then the kind of pain I felt, say, during childbirth."

"Yeah. That pain meant new life. It meant a kind of limitless possibility."

"Right," I say. "Pain means different things at different times in your life. And at different times in history." I tell him about Fanny Burney's description of her anesthetic-less mastectomy in the letter to her sister. "Can you imagine?" I ask. "Aside from the fact that her story is both fascinating and horrifying, the thing that stood out for me was how clearly she articulated the way she managed to step into the pain: it was because she believed it was her best chance at staying alive."

Back in the early 1800s, at the time of Fanny's mastectomy, there were concerns that any form of "dulling the senses" with drugs like morphine, alcohol, or ether would reduce a patient's ability to survive a surgical procedure. It was a deep social anxiety that was intimately connected to cultural understandings of the meaning of pain. For many physicians and theologians of the nineteenth century, the attempt to eradicate pain was deemed a dangerous physical and moral hazard. Sensation, any sensation, was *the* critical function of the human body. "To suspend it by artificial agency," wrote one physician in 1851, "is to set at nought the ordinances of nature."

Without pain, how was a person meant to demonstrate their moral strength and religious faith, or be cleansed of sin? Pain was a test, or an opportunity for redemption, for it was through the crucible of suffering that someone could best express their spiritual convictions. This redemptive aspect of pain was seen to be especially critical for the spiritual health of ladies; anxious men, particularly of the Victorian era, worried that without pain's powerful incentive toward Christian goodness, their women might turn a little... wild. Original sin had perpetuated the natural consequence, since time immemorial, of pain in childbirth. Uncomplaining endurance of that pain was the necessary price for Eve's indiscretions. James Young Simpson pioneered the use of chloroform during birth in the mid-nineteenth century, a proposition that, considering these religious beliefs, was met with a great deal of apprehension. "Chloroform," he was informed by one such angsty clergyman, "was a decoy of Satan that would harden society and rob God of the deep earnest cries which arise in times of trouble."

Thankfully Simpson did not endorse this link between suffering and sin, slyly noting that the most virulent objectors to the use of anesthetics during birth were "caustic old maids whose prospects of using chloroform are for ever passed, or . . . some antiquated lady who grieves and grudges that her daughter should not suffer as their mother has [been] obliged to suffer before them."

Toward the early twentieth century, physicians continued to worry that anesthetics and analgesics would create a society that was overly sensitive and lacking in fortitude and self-control. They observed that with the option of lessening or eliminating pain, patients were not only less willing but less able to endure any amount of discomfort. "Even the slightest sensory disturbances seem to have exaggerated importance," wrote the French surgeon René Leriche in the 1930s. "Far more than our ancestors, we try to avoid the slightest pain, however fleeting it is, because we know that we have the means of doing so. And, by this very fact, we make ourselves more readily susceptible to pain and we suffer more. Every time we fix our attention on anything, we become more conscious of it. So it is in the case of pain."

Fanny Burney's letter is an enduring testament to a kind of resilience that seems, from the vantage of the twenty-first century, almost superhuman. How did Fanny do it? Was it as simple as the fact that, for her, the pain of surgery meant survival instead of all its other possible meanings: disfigurement, disability, and death?

"You know, your pain might represent the very real presence of vulnerability and limits in our life, but also, for me at least, it represents your strength," I say now. "You keep getting up every day and moving through it."

"Thanks," Si says. "That's a nice thing to say."

"I'm not saying it to be nice. It's important to remind ourselves that both things are potentially true. Pain means you are vulnerable. But the way you continue to move through it means you are strong. Pain might be the most catastrophic of all your catastrophic injuries. But also, it's your body's loudest expression of the impulse for continual whole-body healing. Maybe we have to embrace the notion that one thing doesn't cancel the other out."

"Agreed," he says.

"Do you think that there was something more than just viewing the pain as necessary to survival that helped Fanny get through her surgery? Do you think it's possible that two hundred years ago people had greater grit than we do today? Are we just a bunch of twenty-first-century softies?"

He shrugs as he turns into a parking lot adjacent to the pot dispensary. "It would be interesting to compare Fanny's worldview to, say, a Millennial's."

I nod. Eli, born at the tail end of this notoriously agitated generation, has assured us that among his peers, suffering from at least two or three disorders is viewed less as a liability and more as the unavoidable condition of being a young human at the dawn of a new century.

"Okay, my lovely partner-in-crime," Simon says, pulling into a wheelchair-accessible parking spot. "This is it. We're here."

Our cannabis dispensary hostess, Roxy, seems proof positive of Eli's assertion. She's about his age and is aglow with youth and beauty: glossy dark hair spun in a fashionable twist, brown eyes twinkling, and rosy cheeks plumping into a warm smile. A silver hoop sparkles in her right nostril, and her ensemble—black shirtdress over colorful tie-dyed tights and bulky combat boots—reminds me of my own teenage fashion.

"How *are* you guys?" she asks, as if we were old friends.

"Great," Simon says. It's the only appropriate answer when faced with such genuine cheerfulness. "We're wondering what you stock that's specific to pain relief."

For the next five minutes, Roxy provides a detailed description of the dispensary's various strains of pot. It's like a waitress reciting the day's specials; once she's started there's no room to interrupt. In this case we're also given a blow-by-blow of Roxy's various maladies. Northern Lights is the strain she uses for her chronic migraines, while Purple Kush is best for her persistent insomnia. For her anxiety disorder, Bubba Kush is hands down the best. Blue Dream is what gets her through her monthly, debilitating menstrual cramps. "This," she says, placing a jar labeled White Widow on the counter, "is the best all-round. Good for everything—especially if you have a busy day ahead of you."

"Huh," I say, an image of Roxy smoking a White Widow spliff with her morning coffee flashing through my mind. True, I am out of touch with pot culture these days, but—the wake-and-bake strategy? It had never seemed particularly suitable for anyone with a busy day ahead.

"Thing is," Simon says, "I have a brain injury. I don't want anything that will make me stoned. I was thinking more about CBD edibles, with maybe a wee kick of THC."

"Okay, yeah," Roxy says, instantly recalibrating her pitch. In a few minutes, based on her knowledgeable suggestions, we have filled a small basket with an arnica, juniper, and marijuana topical cream, a small vial of a dark-green viscous substance described as a combination of high-grade hempseed oil and amber cannabis honey oil, and several packages of CBD/THC gummies.

"Black cherry, raspberry, mango," Simon says, picking his preferred flavors.

"But this over here," Roxy says moving to the far end of the display case. "This is what I think will work best. I get really bad arthritis in my hands from rolling joints. And this is the only thing that helps."

Simon looks up at me, lips pressing together. *I get really bad arthritis in my hands from rolling joints.*

"C'mon," I say brusquely, pushing the wheelchair toward Roxy. If I look at him a second longer, both of us will bust out in uncontrollable giggles like a pair of stoned teenagers.

"They're suppositories," Roxy says. Simon clears his throat, swallowing down another round of giggles. I don't dare glance at him.

"Suppositories?" I say. "*Anal* suppositories?"

"Yeah. What's great about them is that you can get more of the good-for-pain-relief THC, but you don't tend to get the high feeling. Just a nice relaxed body buzz," Roxy explains, unfazed by my incredulity. She pulls a bag of gel capsules out and plops it on the counter. "I wouldn't use them if you have a busy day planned, but they are great, say, at bedtime."

"Okay," Simon says, grinning. "Sold."

"THEY SHOULD GET LEON PHELPS, aka the Ladies Man, to do some promo for them," Simon says as we exit the store. His voice takes on the lisping lasciviousness that the actor Tim Meadows employed for his recurring character on *Saturday Night Live*, delivering one of Leon Phelps's signature taglines: "Might I suggest... the Butt."

Both of us laugh. That is, until I realize there's an RCMP car parked directly out front of the store. Ridiculously, I lower our brown paper bag filled with cream, oil, edibles, and suppositories down to my side, as if I could hide what we were so obviously purchasing. The officer inside the car is wearing aviators and his inscrutable gaze follows us as we pass by.

"Po-po," I say.

"Be cool," Simon says. "Cannabis is legal. He's not going to do anything."

He doesn't.

"What about the suppositories," I say, as we wait for the van's side door to open and Simon's ramp to unfold onto the asphalt. "Legal, or not?"

Si shrugs, then rolls up the ramp's steep incline. "They're probably not on the current list of government-approved products. But it doesn't matter. The cops don't care about us. It's the unlicensed dispensaries that will be in trouble."

"Good," I say, climbing into the passenger seat. "I don't have the nerves for criminal activity."

"Lightweight." Simon pulls into traffic just as the officer opens his car door and steps out. From the rearview mirror, I watch as he moves toward the door of the dispensary, then the road curves to the left and he disappears.

"Shit," Si says. "I sure hope Roxy has all her paperwork in order."

# 16

# U-Dream

JUNE 12, DAY 325.

Simon deems the trip to the dispensary a success. The edible products are marginally more effective than his prescribed cannabinoid spray, Sativex, and it's easier to manage his dose. He's yet to experience the uncomfortable feeling of being stoned that he sometimes gets with the pharmaceutical spray. And he's used them regularly: there's only one more suppository left and a couple of packs of gummies. The jar of cream is more than half full, but that's because Simon is deeply suspicious of its scent. One of the consequences of his head injury was a total loss of his sense of smell. In the last few years, he's noticed what he calls "whispers of smells" returning, but they are often distorted and inaccurate. Once, driving through a cloud of skunk spray, he smelled ammonia. The one smell he can reliably identify is simmering onions, but then again, to him, a lot of things smell like onions: cooking fish, his own sweat, smoke from winter chimneys. So, for all things olfactory, he relies on me for feedback.

"Tell me honestly," he said one night, sniffing the jar in vain. "If you were to name the fragrance, what would you call it? *Seth Rogen's Armpit*?"

"Maybe," I said, "*Old Hippie* wouldn't be bad either."

"Great." He screwed the lid on decisively and pushed the jar to the back of his bedside table drawer.

Over the past few weeks, with the help of the suppositories in particular, Simon has reduced his hydromorphone use by two milligrams—a small amount, but progress. Still, we wonder if the dispensary products are worth the expense—an expense we have to cover, whereas the costs of the prescribed spray, and the opioids, are covered by workers' compensation.

An unexpected answer to our dilemma arrives in the form of a mason jar full of a grass-colored oil delivered by one of Simon's longtime guitar students, Tom.

"Marie and I thought you might like to try this," he says, handing over the jar. Both Tom and his wife are exceptionally talented songwriters and gardeners. And Marie has discovered an innovative way to transform her organically grown cannabis plants into oil, one that doesn't involve heat. Their suspicion that her cold-press process had produced a unique product was confirmed when they sent the oil to be analyzed by an independent lab. The results were intriguing: tests confirmed her oil contained an exceptionally high amount of THCA, a compound distinct from both CBD and THC that combines the benefits most appealing to Simon: it's anti-inflammatory, which helps with pain like THC, but, like CBD, it lacks a psychoactive component, so it doesn't produce a "high" feeling. Usually THCA is obtained by juicing cannabis leaves, which is inordinately time-consuming and costly. Marie doesn't juice the plants, but her process remains a mystery: her own secret recipe.

"It's the best of both worlds," Tom says of her oil, in his typically understated way. "Keep it in the fridge, though.

Left too long at room temperature, it converts to THC and might make you feel stoned."

The effects of this new oil are not dramatic but rather cumulative. "It's great," Simon says, after ten days. "I can take a teaspoon at bedtime and it helps that difficult transition from sitting in the wheelchair to lying in bed. And I've cut my hydromorphone down by another two milligrams."

When the jar starts to empty, Simon calls Marie to ask if he can purchase another.

"Well, no. I can't sell it under the new legalization regulations," she says. "But we've got a good supply. We'll share what we've got with you."

"Okay," Simon says. "Solid. And—in totally unrelated news—let Tom know that going forward I will be renegotiating his music lesson fee to zero dollars a session."

"Sweet," Marie says. "That's a good deal."

HYDROMORPHONE HAS NEVER helped Simon that much. "It doesn't take the pain away," he says. "It just, for a little, takes me away from the pain." He has identified two key benefits from his opioid use. The first is the small measure of control it provides. "I know it's not giving me lasting pain relief, but if I'm up in front of an audience playing guitar, at least I know I can take a pill and it will help me manage the next hour," he says. "Also, I do think it helps me sleep."

This, we decide, is our next tactic. Marie's THCA oil is helping Simon make the transition from wheelchair to bed. Would a sleep aid help him to further reduce the hydromorphone? He consults with Dr. Jaschinski, and in short order a prescription for the sleeping pill zopiclone is delivered to the house. But Si immediately has second thoughts.

"It's one more thing to be dependent on," he says.

"But maybe it's better than hydromorphone. If you're going to be dependent on something, then at least it should work, and if that something isn't stopping the pain, at least it could be helping you get a good night's sleep."

Still Simon waffles. I suggest picking up an herbal sleep aid instead, and he jumps at the idea. The cashier at my favorite pharmacy suggests a product called U-Dream.

"People love it," she says. "It really works."

Simon tries it midweek and—wow. Late into the night, I lie beside him listening to the beautiful snores. I can't remember the last time this has happened. For years, pain had left him lingering in the shallows of sleep, always on the verge of troubled wakefulness.

"It's powerful," he says the next morning. "I shouldn't take it every night."

So he waits four more nights to take a second U-Dream. Once again he falls asleep quickly, big, breathy snores rattling the air. Peacefulness descends like a weighted blanket, a kind of magical state of grace. The next morning, I wake a few hours before him and am writing in my office when he rolls out of the bedroom.

"Kara?"

"Morning," I say, preoccupied with wrestling a sentence into submission. "How'd you sleep last night? That U-Dream really knocked you out."

"Yeah," he says. "I don't know what to say, but... the pain is gone."

"What?" I leave my desk and kneel in front of his wheelchair.

"I'm kind of scared to talk about it. But it's gone. All gone. Like, usually, even when it's not flaring it's always there, buzzing and crackling like a fluorescent light about to die.

It's an ever-present white noise in my body. And this morning it's not there. No flares; no white noise. It's gone."

"Okay," I say, and start to cry.

"It's okay," Simon says. "Go back to work. Let's not talk about it. I'm going to make myself toast and coffee. Let's see how long it lasts."

"Okay," I say.

Simon hovers within this pain-free window for a few glorious hours, then slowly, over the course of the afternoon, the pain returns to its usual levels. Later, he takes a third U-Dream and has another deep sleep, but the magic doesn't repeat itself the next morning. Still, we are elated. It's the first time in ten years that Simon has experienced substantial pain-free moments. We didn't know if it was possible, and now we do.

At the end of the week, Simon has a consult with Rhonda Wilms. U-Dream is the first thing we discuss.

"Hmmm," Dr. Wilms says. "I'm familiar with U-Dream. And while I am so happy for you, I urge you to be cautious. I don't know what's in that product."

"I do," I say, prepared for this moment with a printout of the herbal ingredients. "There's passionflower, L-tryptophan, and curcumin—"

"No, no," Dr. Wilms interrupts. "That's not what I mean. I know what they *say* is in the product. It's what they're *not* saying that concerns me."

"You think there's something *else* in there," I ask. "They couldn't do that, could they?"

"Sorry, guys," Dr. Wilms says. "Something wacky is going on with that product. The effects are *too* strong. I don't want to ruin the moment for you, but, look, if you notice any neurological issues, stop taking it immediately."

"Well," Simon says, "pardon my French, Rhonda, but... fuck. Fuck fuck fuck."

"Yep," Dr. Wilms says.

IN PAIN RESEARCH LITERATURE, there are many references to *optimal,* or *appropriate,* pain relief. What's rarely discussed is that these designations—optimal, appropriate—are not fixed; like the experience of pain, they're an eternally moving target, constantly being redefined not only by medically sanctioned prescribing guidelines but by cultural, political, and economic forces. The critical question for many—most—medical researchers and practitioners is one of risk versus benefit: How do you provide the greatest pain relief with the fewest side effects? But, especially within a poorly regulated, capitalist economic framework, some within that same community ask a different, deadlier, question: How much money can be made by exploiting suffering people?

In 1810, wine cordial was deemed appropriate pain relief for Fanny Burney's anesthetic-free mastectomy. In the second half of the century, however, there was an explosion of opium-based patent medicines, such as Mrs. Winslow's Soothing Syrup, prescribed by doctors and marketed as a miracle cure for a variety of conditions: headaches, respiratory ailments, diarrhea. It was useful, too, in relieving menstrual cramps and soothing fretful children. Such broad application had a predictable result: people who took the miracle drug because doctors and ad campaigns assured them it was safe to do so became dependent. The stock figure of a typical "dope fiend" emerged in the early twentieth century: weak-willed, self-indulgent, mendacious, depraved—an unproductive and treacherous burden placed on the hardworking members of society. Legislation like the

U.S. Harrison Narcotics Tax Act of 1914 laid the groundwork for police to begin arresting doctors for prescribing opiates. Fearing prosecution, doctors stopped prescribing the drug, and people who had become dependent suddenly no longer had legal recourse to it. Instead, when they turned in desperation to comparable illegal products, they were stigmatized, marginalized, and criminalized.

If that sounds like an eerily familiar narrative, that's because it is. Historically, companies such as Purdue Pharma have recognized that there is big money to be made from exploiting desperation and pain. Purdue, in what surely will go down as one of the most nefarious and deadliest cons in history, established a new industry standard for how to rebrand and market pain medication when they introduced a new drug called OxyContin. In the process, the company made a lot of money and devastated countless lives.

Purdue positioned OxyContin (like Mrs. Winslow's Soothing Syrup) as a safe and effective panacea for a variety of issues: bad backs, knee strain, tooth extraction, headaches, fibromyalgia, sports injuries, and broken bones. The problem? The claims Purdue made weren't true. As early as 1999, a Purdue-funded study of headache sufferers put the OxyContin rate of addiction not at 1 percent, as was so often repeated to patients and doctors, but at a much higher 13 percent. And while perk-based marketing strategies were commonplace in the pharmaceutical industry, it was the first time they were used to market a federally designated Schedule II drug, one deemed to have medical use but with a high potential for abuse. Purdue wasn't using branded merchandise giveaways to pitch an anti-inflammatory that would help you get back out on the dance floor. They were hawking a drug that was almost a molecular identical twin to heroin.

As marketing strategies go, it was fantastically successful: in 1997 there were 670,000 oxy prescriptions for chronic pain filled in the U.S.; five years later, in 2002, that number rose to 6.2 million. Across North America, there was a huge cultural shift in the prescribing of OxyContin, as well as other forms of opioids, for a wide variety of problems. Patients, as consumers within the health care system, could demand access to what was now deemed *appropriate* pain relief.

The massive success of pharmaceutical companies like Purdue was in part based on their ability to exploit the divisive nature of American politics. Co-opting the language of left-leaning pain advocates, pharmaceutical sales reps claimed that all felt pain was real pain and presented themselves as being on a righteous campaign to end suffering. According to these pharmaceutical companies, however, the remedy for suffering was to allow private enterprise—their private enterprise—to provide a solution, ideally with as few troublesome federal regulations as possible, and this was a solution that appealed to those whose politics leaned to the right. If people's pain was being recognized and treated, Democrats were happy; if that treatment didn't involve dipping into a taxpayer's wallet, Republicans were happy. For a short while, Big Pharma made sure everyone was happy.

Are you a time-strapped general practitioner, desperate to provide succor for some of your most demanding, hurting patients? Are you a person-in-pain whose condition threatens every domain of your life, and who, critically, must find a way to get back to work and make money? Are you a big insurance company that, despite the strong body of evidence supporting multidisciplinary clinics as the best type of intervention, will only cover claimants for the cost of a prescription? Do you belong to a twenty-first-century North American culture where being pain-free is viewed as not just a biological imperative but also a critical social entitlement? A drug like OxyContin—pitched as being fast, effective, and most important, relatively risk-free—was the ideal solution. That is, until people whose original complaint was often as non-life-threatening as a sore low back or a torn rotator cuff began to die of overdoses in numbers that exceeded deaths due to car crashes.

The Centers for Disease Control and Prevention estimates that in the U.S., between 1999 and 2020, there have been approximately 564,000 overdose deaths from opioids, both prescription and illicit, although the number is likely much higher as overdose deaths are notoriously underreported. In 1888, the American doctor Silas Weir Mitchell had warned that addiction would increase, not lessen, pain. The last twenty years have provided a potent reminder of this fact: opioids, in many instances, are more likely to protract or exacerbate a chronic state of pain than to solve it.

The word *quackery* is too kind, too quaint, to describe the devastation wreaked by the criminal actions of these pharmaceutical companies. The human cost of their cashed-up mega-manipulations is mind-boggling. In addition to the hundreds of thousands of opioid overdose deaths in the U.S., Canada, and around the world, countless lives have been ravaged, lost to years of substance use disorders. Families have been torn apart. And an essential trust has been obliterated. When people-in-pain enter the medical system, they are often experiencing the most vulnerable and difficult days of their lives. Trust is required to form a healing relationship with a medical practitioner, and for many this trust has been damaged.

Purdue Pharma has been sued thousands of times since it released OxyContin and has repeatedly pled guilty to charges of misbranding, acknowledging that OxyContin had been marketed with the intent to mislead and defraud. In the wake of these multiple class-action lawsuits, the cultural sea change has been reversed, and the prescribing pendulum has swung in the opposite direction. Because many doctors are now hesitant to prescribe opioids, patients who may benefit from them are denied access, while others who have developed a dependence on a drug they were told was relatively risk-free are stigmatized as addicts. And for many of these patients, the underlying pain that prompted them to seek help from the medical system in the first place has yet to be adequately addressed. This combination of untreated pain and opioid dependency, or misuse, is a recipe for blind desperation, potentially leading patients to search out illegal, often unreliable or toxic black-market drugs. And so the deaths by overdose, unintentional or otherwise, continue to multiply.

The objective distance provided by history brings some welcome clarity on the age-old question of risk-versus-benefit when trying to determine optimal pain relief. Anesthetic-free amputations like the one Fanny Burney endured? Those are clearly not a good thing. Pacifying young children with the opium-laced Mrs. Winslow's Soothing Syrup? Also clearly not advisable. Having equitable global access to a safe supply of morphine, or morphine derivative, to treat acute or extreme end-of-life pain? That is a very good goal. But fabricating or misrepresenting data in a massively funded market strategy to oversell a potentially addictive drug is an act of criminal intent. These are relatively straightforward judgments to make, yet the decision to prescribe (or to take) opioids is complex. It should be. It is, and will continue to be, a discussion that Simon and I have with his key physicians. Over the past year, through our continuing conversations, Simon and I have concluded that at some point in his future, the use of stronger opioids—an increase in his hydromorphone, say, or even a switch to oxycodone—might be necessary to provide adequate pain management. We're both thankful that he hasn't reached that place yet. And, for the time being, he will continue to try to reduce his hydromorphone dose, grateful that we have access to Tom and Marie's organic THCA oil as well as the opportunity to invest in the low-risk but time-consuming interventions of pain education, movement, and mindfulness.

But we're soon dismayed to discover that this doesn't mean we can stop being vigilant in investigating the claims of pharmaceutical companies.

ON A RECENT HIKE with my friend Anna, I found myself once again on the verge of tears as I described the amazing morning-after-U-Dream experience.

"No pain," I said. "For the first time in more than ten years. It was like a miracle."

Anna knew the product. Her brother, navigating his own calamitous health crisis, had been having trouble sleeping and swore by the stuff. Now, a week later, Anna, never one prone to small talk, doesn't even say hello when I pick up the phone.

"I have terrible news," she says. "Both the FDA and Health Canada have recalled U-Dream. It has something called zopiclone impurity 22 in it. It's like the prescription drugs zopiclone and eszopiclone, but not quite the same. Maybe it's more potent and addictive? No one seems to know. Health Canada got suspicious when people started reporting unusual side effects, like symptoms of withdrawal and dependence. It's totally creepy. The company—Biotrade—says they have *no idea* how this analogue zopiclone got into their product. Which is insane."

"How the hell does that happen?"

"Right? Hopefully there will be an investigation. I called my bro to tell him. Guess what his reaction was? He bought up all the packages of U-Dream he could get online."

"Shit," I say. "I have to go tell Si."

"SHIT," SIMON SAYS. I follow him as he rolls into the bedroom, picks up the almost full package, and moves toward the garbage pail.

"Wait a sec," I say. "This product is the *one* thing that has given you demonstrable results in the past ten years. Dr. J already prescribed you zopiclone. Maybe it's not so bad. You could just hang on to this package until it runs out."

"Are you nuts? Hiding a potentially addictive drug in a so-called herbal product? What kind of company does that? It's a total betrayal of trust."

"Yes, but—"

"No buts. Whatever this zopiclone impurity 22 is, it's not properly regulated. You heard Dr. Wilms... she was worried about neurological issues."

"You're right, of course," I say. "It's just heartbreaking."

"You're telling me, sister," Si says, dropping the U-Dream package into the garbage.

# 17

# Step Five

JUNE 17, DAY 330.

It's Simon's birthday. He's forty-nine today.

"And boy, do I feel mid-century," he says. "This getting older is not for the faint of heart. Maybe we should talk about the Raptors instead." A few days ago, for the first time in the franchise's history, the Raptors won the NBA finals, and Simon's euphoria has yet to wear off.

We've taken the day to do something rare: eat a picnic lunch on the pier in Gibsons. It's a deluxe spread—kale coleslaw, cornbread, smoked wings, watermelon lemonade, almond cream tart for dessert—and we eat leisurely. It's warm and windy out on the water, silver sun glinting on the cresting waves.

"We should do this more often," I say. "Get out of the house with no other purpose than doing something out of the ordinary. And fun."

Simon nods. "Let's make that part of the TACKLING PAIN protocols: once a month, lunch out."

As we approach a full year of our project, our days have finally found a comfortable rhythm. Si is maintaining a daily twenty minutes on the Dreampad. He does three to five meditation sessions on the iom2, swims for fifteen minutes at least twice a week, does his qigong almost daily, and we squeeze in a roll-walk with Chico in the forest once a week. We still run the peppermint diffuser at night, and I often hurl out double-digit multiplication questions—*what's thirty-two times seventy-eight?*—to help ease Si out of a nighttime spike of pain. With the addition of the CBD pills and the THCA, he's managed to cut his hydromorphone use almost in half, to about ten milligrams every day. His overall pain isn't noticeably less, but our shared sense of agency is at an all-time high.

"What do you think? Are you almost at the point where you could quit the hydromorphone totally?"

"No," he says. "And we're not even discussing it until after the show."

"Fair enough."

The Vancouver release for the new album *Grooves and Ruts* is less than two weeks away. It's been an enormous amount of work for Simon—mixing and mastering the final cuts, organizing the artwork, and getting the CDs made. And now he—and his perpetually beleaguered nervous system—must face the jittery anticipation of the upcoming show.

"Between getting the band ready and keeping up with even a portion of my TACKLING PAIN stuff—I'm at maximum capacity," he says.

"Let me know what I can do. In the meantime, I've had an idea. Remember we were going to put together a five-step action plan but could only come up with four steps? Well, I thought a good fifth one would be networking. Focus more on the 'social' part of the biopsychosocial nature of pain. Make broader connections outside of the micro-verse of you and me."

Simon nods. Together we put together a short list of innovators working in the fields of patient advocacy, pain research, and clinical practice whom we would love to talk with, and when we return home I send out inquiry emails. The next day, as Simon's band Farm Team assembles for a marathon rehearsal, my inbox fills with a series of encouraging replies.

SIMON'S PHYSICAL LIMITATIONS are challenging and very visible. Like many who live with disabilities, Simon is aware of how these limitations provoke a range of reactions from the world around him: many people are sympathetic, some are shocked and saddened, others seem fearful or strangely impatient. Most, I believe, can't imagine what it would be like to live in his circumstances and would be surprised to learn something that for us has become a basic truth: it is pain, that mostly invisible force, and not his physical limitations that has the greatest impact in his daily life. A recurring theme in our conversations is the gratitude we feel to be relatively financially stable. We're far from wealthy, but that's okay. It's stability—and time—that we need to undertake our TACKLING PAIN project. Both of us are horrified by the thought of someone experiencing similar chronic pain while navigating adversarial health and social care systems in an attempt to secure desperately needed resources. To get better insight into the scope of that experience, I connect first with Joletta Belton, pain advocate and author of the blog *My Cuppa Jo.*

In 2010, Joletta was a paramedic and firefighter working in a busy fire station in Southern California. At thirty-three, she'd worked hard to succeed in a profession that was not always welcoming to women.

"There's a lot of folks who believe women don't belong in the fire service," she says, her friendly, wide-open face smiling at me from my computer screen. We're on a Zoom call, sunshine pouring in through the windows of her home office. "But I loved my job. I loved being strong and fit. A badass."

Firefighting was her chosen career, her identity, her sense of purpose. But all of that changed one day when, returning from a routine call, she stepped awkwardly off the fire engine and felt a twinge deep in her hip. Initially, she wasn't worried. It didn't seem like a big deal. But over the next few months the pain became increasingly worse. She couldn't sit to drive. She couldn't lift her right leg to step onto the fire engine. She could no longer do her job safely and was forced to confront the fact that in her current state she was a liability to herself, her coworkers, and the public. So, she took a worker's comp leave, still certain things would resolve quickly with rest and physical therapy.

Difficult days followed. The pain didn't resolve as expected. In fact, it continued to get worse, dominating every moment of her life. And she was confounded: Why was she failing to get better? "I was worried about the future, about what the injury meant for my career, my life. Was I going to be in this kind of pain forever? Could I survive if I was?" she says. "And all the while I still didn't know why: no diagnosis, no pain education, no effective treatment. No answers at all."

When a battalion chief whom she respected—and who she thought respected her—accused her of malingering, she was devastated. "My depression worsened. My pain worsened. My shame worsened," she says. "It was the abyss."

A surgeon finally made a diagnosis of impingement in the hip, and Joletta underwent surgery. It alleviated the worst of the pain, but not all of it. Still, she began the difficult climb out of that abyss only to find herself caught in a worker's comp nightmare. To be eligible for her financial support, she was given a list of restrictions: no squatting; no sitting for long periods of time; no climbing; no awkward positions; no lifting more than twenty pounds; no running.

"Those *no*'s were insidious. The question became, how could I get well enough to do a tough physical job if I couldn't slowly rebuild my strength?" she explains. "I felt guilty all the time—I wasn't working hard enough, or I was working *too* hard. I was always in the wrong. And all that time I was worried I would be tailed by an investigator who was trying to catch me in an 'awkward position'—whatever that means—all to document any so-called infractions that they could use against me. Basically, to call me a liar and a cheat so that they could deny my claim. That was the most terrifying part! Thinking they might take away support because I was caught squatting to tie my shoe or walking my dog."

This no-win situation was echoed in other areas of her life. She pushed herself to attend a work-related party, a draining endeavor but also an important one: she wanted to remain connected to her firefighting family. But she was once again devastated to learn that simply attending the party was being held against her, proof that her pain was not all that bad. Doctors, too, doubted the severity of her pain when she told them she was managing without opioids. But navigating her crisis without the use of pain medication, if possible, was critically important. She couldn't return to work—the thing she desperately wanted to do—if she required pain medication. And finally, friends confronted her about her decision to post only positive messages on social media. Her desire to remain connected, prescription-free, and positive while navigating intense pain was weaponized against her. The meta-message from multiple sources was clear: to *prove* that she was truly in pain and therefore deserving of supports, she should remain isolated, miserable, and reliant on medications.

Over the course of the next year, she tried to reintegrate back into her working life, performing light duties. Some of her superiors were unsupportive; others went out of their way to help her ease back into the job. But even with support it was a difficult year: "I barely remember any of it, I was in such a fog of pain." She was told that to return to her regular duties as a paramedic and a firefighter, she would need to be 100 percent pain-free.

"At the time pain-free no longer felt possible," she says. She made the decision to take medical retirement. Brutally difficult as this decision was, it proved to be a positive one, allowing her to step outside of a dysfunctional system that seemed guaranteed to lead her down a road to greater disability and dependency. Instead, she began a new chapter in her life.

She went back to graduate school and focused her research in pain science. Like Simon and me, she discovered the work of Lorimer Moseley and David Butler and the Explain Pain series of books. "Finally things started to make sense. Understanding the biopsychosocial nature of pain validated my experience and allowed me to finally move forward. Literally. Learning the science of chronic pain made me realize it was safe to move, and so I started moving more." She laughs. "The irony, of course, is that if I knew then what I know now about the biology of pain, I would have been a better advocate for myself. I would have understood that with support, effective interventions, and time, I likely could have gradually returned to full firefighter duties."

"Do you regret the decision?" I ask.

"That's tough to say. Yes. No. Bottom line was, I needed to stop focusing on changing the pain and start focusing on changing my life. I can't look back and say *what if?* I have to keep moving forward."

It took time, but gradually Joletta's pain did change. "People always ask what was the turning point. The truth is, it's hard to pinpoint just one. Better understanding of pain biology was huge. Also recognizing and addressing past trauma. But so was embracing Buddhist philosophy and reading nineteenth-century writers like Dickens and Tolstoy. Writers have been trying to make sense of human suffering for centuries. Photography—literally looking at the world through a different lens—that was important. Blogging, sharing, connecting: all pivotal. I ended up volunteering for the National Sports Center for the Disabled, providing recovery workouts for people practicing and competing in winter sports. That was big for me too. I had to throw out all my preconceptions around the limitations of disability and what people were capable of. It's been a journey. And all of it is important. There's not one single thing."

Joletta is now the co-chair of the Global Alliance of Partners for Pain Advocacy, an organization founded in the belief that pain patients need to be integral partners in the process of establishing guidelines and protocols for the many pain disciplines: research, education, advocacy, pain management, and clinical practice.

"And it all begins with this crazy, radical thought that when people say they are in pain—we believe them," Joletta says. "Imagine how much time and money—not to mention emotional grief—could be saved if, instead of first questioning or investigating their moral integrity, a person-in-pain was immediately offered pain education resources and support in accessing appropriate interventions."

"Crazy," I say.

"Right?!" she says.

Our hour-long appointment has stretched into a three-hour bonding session. Reluctantly, and with a promise to be in touch soon, we sign off.

"Well, yeah," Si says when I relay the key points of our conversation. "Having pain being acknowledged as real is the most basic precursor to finding any kind of solution. If its existence is doubted or denied, then you've already reached a dead end."

NEXT UP, I TALK WITH Tor Wager, director of the Cognitive and Affective Neuroscience Lab at Dartmouth College. Very early in our pain project, I had avidly followed the research being conducted at CANlab. Like a geeky pain-science fangirl, I read all their publications and tuned into the various podcasts featuring Dr. Wager. CANlab's work was appealing to me for two reasons. First, it seemed unique in the way that its scientific inquiry was explicitly bridging the gap that Simon and I had identified earlier, the one that divided pain into an either-or experience: either, in the medical model, pain was a symptom of an underlying pathology; or, in the non-medical model, pain was largely psychological, construed as a set of perceptions or behaviors. But the point of departure for CANlab's main pain investigations was situated precisely at this intersection: How did the physiological and the psychological interact? This was the question they explored through wide-ranging research projects investigating the effects of thoughts, beliefs, and expectations on the brain, the body, and overall health.

The second reason was more specific. In 2013, Dr. Wager was the lead author on a paper published in the *New England Journal of Medicine* that presented the Neurologic Pain Signature. The NPS, which has since become widely used and studied, offers a detailed neurological snapshot of what occurs in the brain when someone experiences the sensations that accompany evoked nociceptive pain (a nonharmful jolt of electricity, say, or an uncomfortable amount of heat or pressure). Using machine-learning algorithms to analyze fMRI scans, CANlab has successfully gone beyond the scope of traditional neurologic brain-mapping (scans that created a statistical map of the brain by identifying key regions that responded to specific stimuli) to creating a vastly more detailed neurological biomarker that can track pain intensity across a wide range of individuals with about 90 to 95 percent accuracy. As far as objective measurements, it's the gold standard, an alternative to the messy variability of self-report.

When I had first read about the Neurologic Pain Signature, I let myself daydream: how amazing would it be to go to Dartmouth and get a detailed analysis of an fMRI scan of Simon's brain-in-pain? The idea that there could be objective confirmation—proof!—of the intensity of his pain was incredibly compelling.

I admit as much to Dr. Wager when we connect one Tuesday afternoon over Zoom. "But," I also admit, "as our personal project has gone on, I've come to suspect that impulse in myself. Now I'm not so sure—for us—what help an objective measurement might provide."

"Right," Dr. Wager says, nodding vigorously. Although he has been one of the leading voices in pain research for the past two decades, and his impressive list of publications is pages long, in person he doesn't seem much older than the undergraduate student he was twenty-some years ago. He smiles frequently, and his sentences tend to trail off into an easy chuckle. That, and the fact that he spent the first fifteen minutes of our conversation asking me questions both about the TACKLING PAIN project and Simon's injuries, has not only put me at ease but also given me insight into the type of creative and collaborative interactions that must routinely occur at CANlab. "I know you have questions for me." He laughs again. "But let me ask you this first: Is that something you guys encountered? Having Simon's pain invalidated?"

"No, not really," I say, explaining that Simon's pain, while mysterious, has always been acknowledged as real. "Partly, I think that's because his injuries were so catastrophic and his ongoing disability so visible." We briefly discuss how pain syndromes associated with spinal cord injury are complex and may include a messy jumble of nociceptive, neuropathic, and neuroplastic pain. "It makes it complicated," I say.

"Well, and that's it exactly, right? Pain is so many things. You can't have a one-size-fits-all prescription," Dr. Wager says. "There are all kinds of biomarkers in the body—genetic, inflammatory, neurological—and they have multiple uses for a researcher. The big one is, indeed, trying to understand what is driving pain in a causal way. If we can better understand that, then we have a better chance of making an accurate diagnosis. And if we can make an accurate diagnosis, we have a better chance at providing the most appropriate treatment."

"Treat the cause, not the symptom?"

"Yeah, exactly. A great analogy is the difference between viral and bacterial infections. In both cases, you might get a fever, a headache, or a stomachache. But these things—fever, headache, stomachache—mean nothing. They are symptoms. You have to know the underlying cause. If it's bacterial, you treat with antibiotics. If it's viral, you'll take a totally different approach. Of course, it gets more complicated with pain, but our goal is to identify a clear model of how the brain constructs these various pain experiences, because if we don't have a way of measuring pain except for self-report, treatments tend to be based on symptoms."

CANlab's research clearly demonstrates that there are multiple pathways that contribute to the pain experience, once again underscoring the fact that pain always has a context. Analysis of a vast array of fMRI scans has clearly demonstrated that different kinds of pain arise from different sources in the brain.

"Is it this pathway? Or that pathway? Or is it *all* the pathways?" Dr. Wager says. "If we can continue to refine our ability to identify these different pathways, we can refine our ability to assess and treat. Is surgery indicated? Or pharmaceuticals? Or would a combination of physical therapy and psychological intervention be more appropriate?"

"Are you able to make those determinations now?" I ask.

"No. Not yet. Not reliably person-to-person. Right now, the scan works pretty well for evoked pain. But it doesn't work quite so well for other kinds of ongoing pain, or at least the jury is still out. It's hard to study that kind of chronic pain for a variety of reasons." A brief discussion follows as to why this might be so. Evoked pain, Dr. Wager explains, refers to an acute response to pain-inducing stimuli such as pressure, or extreme heat or cold, and as such it's relatively easy to create and manipulate in a lab-experiment setting.

On the other hand, ongoing, real-life pain has a vast array of variables that are difficult to both identify and account for.

However, puzzle piece by puzzle piece, CANlab is starting to build an interesting picture. They've demonstrated, for example, that there are similar but distinct brain pathways for evoked physical pain and for emotional pain, like the kind activated by being socially excluded or rejected. They've shown that adopting a mindfulness approach to pain management can reduce the Neurologic Pain Signature as effectively as a moderate dose of opioids. Unsurprisingly, given his multidisciplinary approach to science, Dr. Wager explains that CANlab will continue to investigate the intersection of multiple systems in the body—the neurological, the endocrine, the immune—and the ways in which all these things may color and shape the experience of pain.

"Inflammation has become a hot topic these days," he says. "It's currently a kind of catch-all term, and really we only have a few measures that are able to track it. But there do seem to be interesting correlations linking inflammation to trauma, pain, depression, chronic illness, and PTSD that are emerging. We likely haven't figured out the best way to measure it yet," he says, laughing. "You could compare inflammation in the body to a jungle. And right now, the only thing we're able to see is bananas."

"But—it's a place to start, right?"

"Exactly."

Talking to Dr. Wager reignites my dream to get a Neurologic Pain Signature scan of Si's brain, but when I ask if the technology will be widely available in the coming years, he shakes his head. Not in the foreseeable future, he explains. Currently the technology is too expensive and complicated for broad use. But he has hope, pointing out how quickly things changed in the world of genetics. Initially the practical application of the technology was incredibly limited. Now, for a couple hundred bucks, anyone can have a genetic workup done.

"Imagine," Si says when I explain about the scan, and the information it could potentially provide, "how much time we might have saved over the last ten years."

"And worry, and risk," I say, thinking about the nerve ablation procedure.

"Even if it was bad news," Si says. "Like there-is-nothing-you-can-ever-really-do-for-this-kind-of-pain news, it's still information I'd like to have."

THE GREAT HOPE of being able to identify biomarkers for pain is that decisions about treatment will be tailored for the individual. But are these research advances being adequately translated into clinical practice? I'm hoping that Hance Clarke, the Knowledge Translation Chair for the University of Toronto Centre for the Study of Pain, can answer that question. He explains that while *patient-centered care* is currently a fashionable phrase in medicine, and conveys an admirable intention, its aim is sadly not always realized.

"The practice of medicine," he says, "has, over the past twenty years, become dominated by an algorithm dogma. We are asked to treat patients based on mean averages from clinical trials, never fully acknowledging that those trials are often carried out on very homogenous populations. But you can't practice pain medicine that way. You *have* to treat the individual person in front of you."

Internationally recognized for his innovations in patient care, Dr. Clarke has an impressive list of credentials. He's a staff anesthesiologist at Toronto General Hospital, where he spearheaded the development of the Transitional Pain Service, the first comprehensive, patient-centered pain care practice that aims to provide timely interventions for people at high risk of developing chronic post-surgical pain. As director of TPS, he has a ridiculously busy schedule, but he graciously agrees to a Zoom conversation on a rare day off.

"So..." I ask, tentatively, uncertain how to properly frame the question, "in your opinion, is a research focus on trying to identify various biomarkers for pain—neurological, genetic, inflammatory—helpful? Or does it exacerbate this kind of dogmatic algorithm-based thinking?"

"Well," he says, "the work that is being done is great, great science. And it is all important, useful information. But the question becomes, what next? What do we do with this information? What happens when you are confronted with an individual person who is in pain? That person often has difficult decisions to make and a difficult journey ahead."

TPS takes a multidisciplinary approach to pain management and reduction, providing individualized support to patients. "The first part of the equation is identifying the surgical patients who are at increased risk," Dr. Clarke explains. Certain types of surgeries are more likely to be associated with post-operative pain, as is any intervention that results in nerve damage. A pre-existing pain condition, current or past substance misuse, and a history of anxiety, depression, or trauma are all complicating factors. If a person is desperately afraid of surgery, has poor social networks, or is unable to halt the merry-go-round of catastrophizing thoughts, they too are at higher risk.

"We've been trying to shift the framework that we practice pain medicine in by acknowledging that no one single intervention, no one single medication, is going to be a magic bullet," Dr. Clarke says. "One of the places medicine has failed is by promising people a cure. The fact is, with certain kinds of injuries there is going to be a certain amount of pain to move through. What we can do is to get the supports in place to navigate that process in a way that is meaningful and useful to the individual patient. Are we able to prevent all chronic pain? No. But we can tackle—and hopefully limit—pain distress and pain disability. And we do that by saying, look, we don't have all the answers, but we do have the resources to help you explore what your brain can do; what exercise can do; what medicine can do."

"One of the reasons we embarked on our project," I explain, "was to recreate, as best we could, what seemed to us a kind of mythic gold-standard multidisciplinary pain clinic for ourselves. But—" I pause momentarily.

"—it's not mythic at all," he says, smiling.

"Right."

As an outspoken national pain and addictions strategist, Dr. Clarke has played a leading role in providing evidence-based information concerning both the risk factors and the misconceptions surrounding opioid use. "Responsible opioid stewardship has become a significant component of the work we do," he explains. A key goal is to never have a patient leave the program on a higher dose of opioids than when they arrived. But this piece of the pain-puzzle is often complicated. "I might see a patient who has had fibromyalgia for twenty years and who manages their day-to-day on high doses of an opioid. Still they are telling me their pain is a ten out of ten. I might then acknowledge that the opioids seem to no longer be providing relief and suggest that we—carefully, slowly, with support and various treatment alternatives—explore a different route. Some people are open to that conversation; some aren't."

The Transitional Pain Service team, with funding from Health Canada, has created a road map for setting up similar services, which is currently being adopted not only across Canada but also in countries as far away as Australia and Norway. A global innovator in pain care services, Dr. Clarke is also leading the charge in another key area that he believes is under-researched: the medical use of cannabis.

"We know that roughly one in five of our patients are using cannabis to self-medicate," he says. "The health care world is extremely dichotomized on the subject. Some believe cannabis will become the next socially sanctioned health risk, like alcohol or tobacco. Others feel it should be, for responsible adults, a legitimate treatment option."

"Has legalization complicated that?"

"In a way, yes," he says. We discuss how the government is now collecting huge tax revenue on cannabis sales. There's no longer much incentive for either the cannabis industry or the government to fund medical research. And so many physicians—without clear guidelines on dosing, or how cannabis might interact with other medications—are reluctant to recommend it. "But now that it is legalized recreationally, people *are* self-medicating, and using cannabis much more frequently," he explains. "Unfortunately now, it's often without the support, or oversight, of a health care practitioner. We could be doing better."

To address this gap, Dr. Clarke has established the Medical Cannabis Real-World Evidence trial, hoping to build a repository of patient data that could help establish a set of best practices for people using cannabis medicinally. After admitting to some of our own self-medicating adventures

(Dr. Clarke is particularly intrigued by the success of the suppositories and Marie's THCA oil), I promise we'll follow up and enroll Simon in the trial.

"Any kind of dosing and product guidelines would be helpful in figuring out what to try next," I say.

"Of course," he says, smiling. "Like all things related to pain, it's a work in progress."

"A WORK IN PROGRESS, indeed," Simon says. It's late and we're snuggled under the covers, Chico snoring softly in his dog bed beside us. Neither of us can fall asleep. Si updates me on the progression of band rehearsals, and I outline my conversation with Dr. Clarke. "Fact is," he says, "I have felt particularly under construction lately."

It's been a rough week, heading into the album release show. Simon's sleep has been splintered and he's fallen back into a familiar cyclical state: more pain equals less sleep equals more worry equals more pain, and so on and on. He had made a decision over the winter to limit gigs, both to let him concentrate on recording the album and to give his nervous system a break from performance anxiety.

"The problem with that," he explains, "is that performing is not like riding a bike. You have to keep doing it consistently to be competent. It's been more than a month since I played live. And taking that break has only made me more nervous heading into this show." He's doubled down on all his TACKLING PAIN strategies, adding as much Dreampad time in a twenty-four-hour period as he can, but he's becoming increasingly frustrated at how ineffective it suddenly all feels. "I'm spitting in the wind," he says.

"Well, we know none of our strategies are quick fixes. We know none of them alone can guarantee complete success," I say. "But they are things you do repeatedly over a long period, hoping that the small moments of grace—like the one you had on the morning after taking the U-Dream—happen more frequently. It's a harm-reduction strategy. You know, things might be even worse if you weren't doing all this work."

"It's hard to imagine it being worse."

"Let's just take it one step at a time. *Keep on doing first things first*," I say, quoting his own song lyrics to him.

Simon nods.

"You're ready. You've got a great band, great songs, a great venue. The show is going to be great. I'm looking forward to it for the both of us."

"Thanks," Si says. "I appreciate that. But I think the most positive thing I can say right now is that at least this time next week, it will all be over."

# 18

# A Night at the Cultch

JUNE 29, DAY 342.

Herbie Hancock is playing at the Queen Elizabeth Theatre, a marquee show for the Vancouver International Jazz Festival. All day long Simon has been receiving texts from musician friends apologizing for not attending his album release party. Tonight, they are all going to see Herbie.

"It's entirely possible we might play to an empty theater," Si says as Jay, Boyd, Paul, and I unload the equipment, piling instruments, amps, guitar stands, and drums in the cramped parking space behind the Cultch. The late afternoon sun casts a honeyed glow over the spring vegetation—dusty leaves of purslane, plantain, dandelions—that thrive in the graveled edges of a laneway in northeast Vancouver. Otherwise known as the Vancouver East Cultural Centre, the Cultch houses a beautiful theater and gallery space.

"Let's hope not!" says a voice from the back door. It's Yuri, the event organizer. He's the program director at Kickstart, an organization that supports and promotes artists within the disability community. It's the first time Simon has partnered with them and, so far, it's been amazing. Yuri—who appears to have boundless energy—has done the difficult and generally thankless work of booking the venue, hiring a sound engineer, and promoting the show, leaving Simon able to focus solely on rehearsing. It's a rare and wonderful occurrence, and I only wish Simon could enjoy it more. But today, when I asked him on the drive over what he was feeling, his answer was unequivocal: dread. Utter and total dread.

"It's Herbie Hancock, man," Si says as we all follow Yuri into the building. "Who could begrudge the city of Vancouver if they chose his show over mine?"

"Pfffft!" Yuri waves his hand over his shoulder, dismissing the notion. "That's nerves talking."

"Yes, sir," Simon says with mock seriousness as Yuri leads us through the backstage wings and onto the empty stage. Ascending rows of empty chairs stare back at us, and the air smells softly of sawdust. "It's true: I am definitely entering the full-on imposter syndrome phase of pre-performance preparation. Shit! That's a lot of seats."

A small elevator leads to a green room area, where the wheelchair-accessible washrooms even contain accessible showers. And there's a kitchenette stocked with water, tea, coffee, wine, and beer.

"Not only can I use the washroom, I can have a shower, if I wanted," Simon says. "Not that I want to but, wow, does that ever make me happy."

"Right?" Boyd says. "It's as if the blueprints of this place set out to include wheelchair users from the get-go. Imagine that!"

We head back downstairs, and Yuri leads me to a table in the lobby designated for merchandise. I'm printing out a small sign—*CDS $15*—when there's a knock at the front entrance. It's Emily, Simon's sister. She's flown in from Toronto this afternoon to see the show.

I yelp, gesture an exuberant hello, and run off to find Yuri, who has the keys to the front doors.

"I can't believe you're actually *here*," I say, after we've hugged. "Let's go see Simon."

In the theater, sound check isn't going well. Simon, Jay, Boyd, and Paul have been joined by the fifth member of the band, the loveable piano, accordion, and trumpet player Walter Martella. The setup looks great, with a wall-sized image of the album cover providing a backdrop to the band. But something is wrong. Brows are furrowed. Frustration clips and hardens consonants when anyone speaks. The entire band is squaring off with the sound man, who is currently invisible to Emily and me, a disembodied voice booming from the sound booth. There are problems with the monitors, the onstage amps that allow the band members to hear one another, and Paul, generally so easygoing, tugs on the visor of his baseball cap with open irritation as he challenges the sound man's assertion that everything should be fine now.

"Ah, no," he says. "It's not."

Simon is unusually quiet as he fusses with the dials on his amp, his face a blank mask of settled tension. But—the instant he sees Emily—he smiles. "We should be done here in half an hour," he says, waving from the stage. "Maybe forty minutes. Then I can give you a proper hug."

We give him a thumbs-up and exit the theater. I look at my watch: two hours until the doors open to the public.

"Hungry?" I ask.

"Always," Em says.

We take a circuitous route, wandering through residential streets, slowly making our way to Commercial Drive. We talk fast, catching each other up on our lives, bumping shoulders as we walk. Along the Drive we pass espresso bars and bakeries, considering Thai, then Mexican, takeout, finally opting for a few large pizzas.

"You guys should be really proud of the album," Emily says.

"I am," I say. But, because it's Em, I allow myself to admit a thought that has long gone unsaid. "I don't know if we'll be able to do it again. I don't know if we should."

As much fun as making the album has been, it's also been stressful, and I see, more than ever, how limited Simon's resources are to cope with that extra stress. Tonight is a good example. In the not-so-distant past, playing big audiences at festivals would psych him out a bit. A reasonable amount. He'd be extra nervous. But an opportunity like that was also fun, exciting. A novel experience, a chance to break out of constantly playing the barroom scene. It would be something to celebrate and enjoy. But here we are, in this gorgeous theater, with logistical and financial support from Kickstart, and he's playing his original music with an incredibly talented and supportive band of musicians whom he loves and admires. It's the dream, really. But he can't feel anything but total dread. And it's not that he's not aware of, and hugely grateful for, all those things. He is. But even after a year of all our strategies to tackle pain, he's still at a tipping point in his nervous system where more anxiety means only one thing: more pain.

"Playing live is costing him too much right now," Emily says.

"Exactly. Pain has him running at a constant deficit. We've haven't been able to shift it that much." I sigh, realizing that this is the first time I've allowed myself to say it out loud. "It's a conundrum. Music is the thing that Simon has worked at all his life. The thing that's most meaningful to him. He fought so hard to return after his accident. And… he's good at it. Really good."

Emily gives my hand a squeeze as we reach the theater.

"So… it feels impossible to not keep playing live," I continue. "But like this? It also feels unsustainable."

Sound check, thankfully, is over. Yuri joins us in the elevator up to the green room, where Simon, Boyd, and Walter are practicing vocal harmonies. Emily leans in to hug Simon.

"Ticket sales have been hopping. It's going to be a full house tonight," Yuri says. Over Emily's shoulder, Simon's face blanches. I decide to go pure Pollyanna.

"That's amazing," I say, depositing the pizzas on the counter. Simon nods but doesn't say anything.

Yuri returns to the box office, the guys resume their singing, and Emily and I retreat to the kitchenette. We forgo tea in favor of a beer for her and a glass of wine for me.

"I see what you mean," Em says quietly. "Si's *nervous*."

"Right?" I say. "But the crazy thing is, I know it's going to be a great performance."

"Well," she says, raising her bottle to clink my glass. "At least *we* can enjoy the show."

The stage manager pokes her head out of the elevator to announce that the doors will open in five minutes, then disappears. All five noisy musicians pause as they collectively inhale. Then exhale. "I think," Paul says, breaking the silence, "we should open with 'Sweet Melinda.'"

Another long pause swells before Simon responds with a drawn-out *hmmmmm.* He's been planning on playing the entire album in order. "Sweet Melinda" comes second, so it's not a big change; he could simply flip tracks one and two. But "Sweet Melinda" is a tough song to play first: it's quiet and precise and requires him to execute a complex picking pattern that's hard to manage when navigating opening-song jitters. To an outsider, this type of decision may seem minor, but it isn't to Simon, especially so close to curtain time. Still, he has implicit trust in Paul's instincts.

"Okay," he says, looking as if he might puke. "Let's do it."

I lean over and give him a kiss. "Em and I are going downstairs to man the CD table. We'll see you on the other side."

"Where there will be club sandwiches, chicken wings, and beer on tap," Emily says.

"Hallelujah."

I give him one more kiss. "Merde," I whisper in his ear, the dancer's equivalent of *break a leg.*

IT WAS A GOOD CALL, starting with "Sweet Melinda." And right from the opening notes, it's not just an amazing night of music; it's magical. As part of Kickstart's mandate to make the arts more accessible for both disabled performers *and* spectators, Yuri has hired two women to sign the lyrics. They stand behind Simon, their hands and bodies performing a complicated and beautiful dance of embodied sound. Somehow, *seeing* the music this way—negotiated through the expressive gestures of sign language—enhances it in ways I could never have imagined.

The guys are on, but it's not just that. It's also the theater. I've seen the band play outdoor events where some of the intimacy of the quieter songs is lost in the large open space. I've also seen them play intimate cafés where the rockiness of the louder songs is difficult to contain. But this midsized theater with its black walls, sawdust air, and attentive audience? It's the perfect size to house Simon's songs, feeling both intimate and spacious, and all the musicians—veteran improvisers—respond at once. The songs are transformed into something brand new, even to me.

Peppered throughout the audience are many beloved faces. Poet Michael Barnholden, who cowrote three of the album's songs, is in the front row with his wife, Nancy Newman. And Eli, who snuck in just before the show started, is sitting next to them with his roommate, Robin. I'm thankful that they, along with Emily, are here, because tonight the audience has become an integral part of the performance. The exhale of our response after a particularly powerful song, that *whoosh* of communal feeling that heralds wild applause—it's all become part of the music.

The last set ends with a handful of covers: Taj Mahal's "Corinna"; Dylan's "Crash on the Levee"; Bowie's "Moonage Daydream." At the back of the theater, Emily and I get up to dance. The room is suffused with so much raw joy that it becomes a kind of physical force, or connective tissue, one that links all our beating hearts. If only it were possible to bottle this communal joy into something Simon could dab behind his ears or pour into a shot glass as a remedy for the exhaustion, pain, and anxiety that inevitably precedes moments like these.

"HOW ARE YOU FEELING?" I ask at the end of the night as we drive back, bone-tired, to the hotel room.

"Happy," he says. "Sad. It was a great night, better than I could have imagined. But I don't know if I'll ever be able to rally the energy to do it all over again." He sighs. "I love you, Stanley. And I love playing music. But tonight might have been my performing curtain call."

# 19

# A Question As Yet Unanswered

JULY 18, DAY 361.

"I don't have words anymore. It is what it is," Si says. He's talking on the phone, and although I'm only privy to one side of the conversation, it's clear his dad has been inquiring about a particularly bad pain spike in the last twenty-four hours. "Today the pain keeps asking questions, ones I can't answer." Simon pauses, then adds: "At least not yet."

It strikes me that with this new metaphor—pain as an unanswered question—we've come full circle, returning back over ten years ago to the frightening first days of extreme pain, when the unanswered question was urgent: *What the hell is wrong?* That sounds depressing, but it isn't, really. In fact, Simon's new metaphor is one of the most grounded things I've heard him say all year.

It is commonly accepted that metaphors are important in art and literature. But metaphors are critically important in all domains of human interaction that require complex ideas or experiences to be translated into a common and accessible language. Metaphors in literature are understood to be decorative, figurative—that is, less concretely real—and their abstract truth is something we intuit rather than reason out. Metaphors move through us, like a river current, or a piece of music, invisible waves transfiguring our thoughts and emotions. We accept this kind of literary metaphor as something quite different from the metaphors used by the medical community to describe things as complex, say, as pain. Medical metaphors, deeply embedded in an edifice of scientific authority, are often mistakenly perceived as unassailable fact and granted the weight of objective truth—even though what they more accurately represent is science's best-guess theory of the time.

Descartes's theory of pain perception was expressed in metaphorical terms when he asserted that the transmission of pain from the site of injury to the pineal gland inside the brain was similar to the act of pulling on a cord that rang a bell at the opposite end. While the ringing of a bell was a metaphor that would have been accessible to his seventeenth-century audience, it didn't fully reflect Descartes's complicated thinking on the topic of pain. But this basic mechanistic metaphor formed the conceptual foundation for the following four centuries of research and medical practice, going relatively unchallenged until Patrick Wall and Ron Melzack replaced the bell with a series of gates—opening the door (metaphorically) for a whole new way of thinking about pain.

All this to say: our metaphoric language matters.

Medical metaphors tend to be mechanistic (pain as a ringing of a bell or an opening and closing of gates) or militaristic, the language of healing strangely muddled with the language of battle. Pain is seen as an enemy, one that needs to be fought and subdued with pain*killers*. Some metaphors reflect our culture's desire that pain be a measurable experience. Pain as *the fifth vital sign* was a slogan trademarked by the American Pain Society and adopted by the U.S. Veterans

Health Administration in 1998. The intention behind this rebranding was deliberate and humane, based in the notion that if pain were routinely assessed along with the other vital signs (pulse, blood pressure, temperature, and respiration), it stood a much better chance of being treated adequately. But functionally, this metaphor falls short. While a doctor can take a temperature or measure blood pressure, there are still no objective ways to measure persistent pain. In the wake of the North American opioid crisis, critics of the slogan blame it for bombarding the medical community and the public with messages that pain is being chronically undertreated, thus contributing to a climate that is vulnerable to the manipulations of companies like Purdue Pharma.

Pain, traditionally, *has* been chronically undertreated, so it's hard to criticize the vital-sign metaphor for drawing attention to that fact. For me, its metaphoric failings are more basic: in its insistence on measuring pain along with the other vitals, it harkens back to the Cartesian biomechanical model that insisted that all *real* pain was locatable and quantifiable. It allows us to avoid investigating the ways in which the experience of pain, the perception of pain, and the concept of appropriate pain relief are not just essential issues of health care but also cultural constructs unique to specific times and places.

And now the World Health Organization has named pain a disease. While this is generally considered progress, there is still some debate about the accuracy of this renaming. Currently, the winning argument is that chronic pain qualifies as a disease of the central nervous system based upon the functional and structural changes that occur in the brain when a pain-state persists for longer than three months. But the counterpoint is that pain-as-disease represents a type of circular thinking that is both semantically and conceptually confusing: How can the symptom "pain" be the cause of a disease also called "pain"? In this counterargument, pain (as an experience, a symptom, a pathology) is viewed as too complex to be reduced to a self-generating state, a symptom that creates its own disease.

Simon and I have mixed feelings on pain-as-disease. As a metaphor, it is powerful, and there are many compelling reasons that it should be promoted. As Nanna Brix Finnerup outlined at the Neuropathic Pain conference, it was hoped that the new definition would promote a more globally uniform understanding of the complex nature of pain, which in turn would decrease stigmatization and promote greater awareness and education.

Pain-as-disease was also meaningful for Simon and me. In the early days, when his pain escalated so dramatically and we didn't know why, our fear that something was wrong was profound. And for good reason—the whole history of human evolution has taught us that, if we want to survive, pain is a problem that needs to be addressed, and quickly. But the stress caused by unexplained and, perhaps, unsolvable pain is one of the key factors that directly contributes to, and can amplify, suffering. We needed the gravity of a word like *disease* to transition us out of the panic into a deeper understanding of how Simon's stressed and injured nervous system was behaving in unreliable ways.

Yet, as our yearlong experiment has progressed, Simon has increasingly said that pain-as-disease is a metaphor that no longer serves him. Like pain as the fifth vital sign, pain-as-disease returns us to a conceptual understanding rooted in a medical domain. It's tempting, of course, to leave it there, because it's simpler to not have to account for the many ways in which the lived experience of pain is influenced, even constructed, by social, political, and economic factors. It's a tough job being responsible for alleviating pain, any kind of pain, but especially the unmeasurable, boundless kind. How much easier it would be to leave it in the hands of the clinicians and researchers, laud them for the success stories, but, more likely, blame them for prescribing either too much medication or too little, and denounce their insensitivity to the plight of their patients when no solution is to be found.

When we insist on metaphors that circumscribe pain as solely a medical issue we are in danger of missing a critical point: when it comes to suffering, it's not just doctors, nurses, therapists, caregivers, and researchers but all of us—individually and socially—who must share that responsibility.

This past year, as Simon and I have grappled with how to conceptualize pain's shifting center, our metaphors have routinely transfigured. At first, Simon's pain was an angry child—Rupert, that snotty asshole. Rupert was an outsider, an invasive, entitled entity that punished Simon with his violent outbursts. But mid-experiment, that metaphor shifted. "Fake news, fake news," Simon would say, talking directly to the blooms and surges and spasms traveling through the paralyzed limbs of his lower body. "Everything is okay, I'm fine, this is just fake news." In this linguistic equation, pain was the ultimate postmodern headline, signifying everything but meaning nothing. Not even Simon's own body was a reliable source of information.

Now we've come full circle, and pain once more is a question as yet unanswered. I like the way this metaphoric construction echoes Patrick Wall's conception of pain as a need state, like hunger or thirst, and that in posing its question it motivates us to take necessary action to ensure our survival. While many in the medical community prefer pain-as-disease—something to be fought, conquered, vanquished—Wall consistently reminded us of the fact that pain is an experience that humbles us all. "I do not believe one can ever be too familiar with pain," he said toward the end of his life as he battled cancer. "It is too deep." This is an astoundingly bold statement from the man who was commonly referred to as the world's leading expert on pain.

Consider this: If birth finds its opposite in death, what is the opposite of life? In the material world, the best contender is pain. As one of humanity's greatest evolutionary gifts to ensure survival, pain insists on bumping us up against the outer edges of our mortality, the precise state that brings us closest to contemplating the great unknowable mystery of what lies on the other side of life. As such, pain is an integral part of a vast and intricately beautiful web of being that connects us to every other living and dying thing—not a condition to be cured.

Understanding, alleviating, accepting, moving through—these all seem like possible worthy goals when confronting pain. But *solving*? *Curing*? After a year of our TACKLING PAIN project, these now seem as impossible as they are unwise.

IT WAS, IN PART, a similar thought that spurred the Vancouver physician Michael Negraeff to create the nonprofit organization Pain BC, an online hub where people-in-pain and their care providers can connect. In 1995, Michael was a young doctor-in-training, finishing up an anesthesiology residency at UBC, when his life took an unexpected turn. On a rare day off, he went skiing on the fabled slopes of Whistler Mountain. It was mid-afternoon when several of the ski lift chairs began to swing erratically. Four chairs, carrying ten people, detached from their lift line and plummeted to the ground below. There was one fatality and multiple injuries. Michael suffered severe trauma to his spinal cord.

"It was T3/T4 complete," he tells me over a Zoom call, employing the shorthand lingo shared by people familiar with spinal cord injury, "complete" meaning that he has no sensation or movement below his T3/T4 vertebrae. "The neuropathic pain was there from day one," he explains. "Buzzing and burning around the level of injury."

Simon and I had first become familiar with Michael's story after reading an article in *The Spin*, a magazine dedicated to people with spinal cord injuries. "There was a moment in the article that really spoke to Simon," I explain. "You were discussing the multitude of things a person needed to address in the aftermath of a serious spinal cord injury to get back to a new normal—mobility, spasms, bowel, bladder, sex, sleep—and saying that, after about the first year, you felt like you were starting to figure all those things out. But when the realization hit that the pain wasn't going away—that was one of the toughest moments."

"Yeah, it was a little like shaking your fists at the universe and saying, 'You've got to be kidding me. This is *too* much. This kind of pain should *not* be part of the bargain.'"

"When Simon read that, he said, 'That's the kind of guy who'd make a great pain doctor.'"

"Well, it's certainly true that my own experience was an influence on pursuing a specialization in pain," he says of his decision, post-medical residency, to complete a fellowship in pain at the Australian and New Zealand College of Anaesthetists. "I wanted to know more. What caused chronic pain? Why did some people get it, and others didn't? And what could we be doing better to help? Chronic pain is like a cake—there's all sorts of layers."

After completing the fellowship, Michael moved back to B.C., taking a position at Vancouver General Hospital, where he found himself immersed in a system in which pain was viewed almost exclusively as a symptom of another illness, never as a problem on its own. "Pain is an orphaned topic, always viewed as a by-product of another, bigger, issue," he says. "But the fact is, chronic pain affects roughly 25 percent of the population—that's more than heart disease, diabetes, and lung disease combined. I started to realize the system needed a fundamental change in how it viewed the problem if we were going to be able to provide better programs that addressed pain, pain-disability, and pain-distress."

The difficult question, of course, was *how?*

Initially Michael imagined more multidisciplinary clinics and more resources dedicated to the issue. But, not surprisingly, there wasn't a readily available pot of money to dedicate to pain.

"Someone recommended that one way to get funding was to create a nonprofit organization," Michael laughs. "I was very skeptical. I had a busy clinical practice; I knew nothing about running an organization. And really, it was the last thing I wanted to do. But then we hired Maria, first as a consultant, and everything changed. We were joined at the hip for six or seven years to make Pain BC a reality."

He's referring to Maria Hudspith, the current executive director of Pain BC, their once fledgling, now flourishing and globally recognized organization. Maria is also the co-chair of the Canadian Pain Task Force, mandated to provide recommendations for a cohesive national pain strategy.

"Maria is amazing," Michael says. "She knows how to bring people together, make connections. Pain BC is successful because of her."

Together they set out a mission statement in line with Lorimer Moseley's prescription: to enhance the well-being of all people living with pain through empowerment, care, education, and innovation. It was critical to them to recognize that none of those things could be accomplished without a fundamental shift in the systems that people-in-pain rely upon.

"When I was approached to work with Pain BC, I was really excited," Maria explains, when she and I sit down to chat. "What Michael envisioned was change at a micro level—impacting an individual person's lived experience of pain—*and* at the macro level—change in how pain is understood within health and social systems of care."

Right out of the gate Pain BC was clearly oriented toward activism, Maria explains. Even though people who routinely face discrimination have much higher rates and severity of chronic pain, previous conversations in Canada had not been attuned to issues of equity and diversity. But Pain BC is unique in integrating the lessons of anti-oppression from the outset.

"We had to," Maria says. "When we started a dialogue with people-in-pain, it was clear that much of the trauma they experienced had happened within the systems meant to care for them. And this, of course, was a huge barrier to healing. That, I think, has been the most radical insight for our entire Pain BC team—many of whom are people who live with persistent pain. Pain is not just a medical issue. It is a social justice issue as well."

It takes less than a minute of conversation for me to be in full agreement with Michael: Maria is amazing. She not only acknowledges the complexity of pain but embraces it, and there is both a fierceness and a generosity in her manner: the ideal combination of traits for an advocate of social change.

"When we started out in 2010, there wasn't a blueprint for what we wanted to do," she explains. "There were a few fledgling peer support groups; there was the International Association for the Study of Pain. But we really wanted to create a movement around the issue. Bring pain out of the shadows and catalyze partnerships with people from various other disciplines. Part of the problem with pain," she says, reiterating Michael's point, "is that it exists everywhere and nowhere at once. We couldn't just say we were going to tackle pain in one specific area, say, the hospital, or long-term care facilities, or in the construction industry." Somehow, the Pain BC team decided, they had to address the big picture. Instead of breaking pain down into segregated silos, they set out to make connections.

"People who take control of managing their own pain have better outcomes," Maria explains. This is why Pain BC started out with what she refers to as bottom-up approaches: interactive online tools meant to support and educate both people-in-pain and their health care providers. Through the establishment of a podcast, a pain support line, and counseling and educational programs, Pain BC has created multiple ways for people to access this support.

"I think these programs have helped to legitimize the issue of pain," Maria says. "And we're starting to see some top-down change too: the federal government actually has a page dedicated to pain on its website, and they have mandated the Task Force to make recommendations for a national action plan."

All this, Maria feels, is going to make a difference. "Over the last ten years there has been a dramatic shift," she says. She describes how Pain BC has recently been contracted by ICBC—the province's main auto insurer—to redesign their process for dealing with pain complaints and to develop staff training programs. "Ten years ago the idea that an insurance agency would contract a chronic pain advocacy organization to develop protocols—that would have been radical. But as we move further away from a model that says to get help for your pain, you first need to prove it, and when we use trauma- and violence-informed approaches to compassionate care, well, there's going to be a sea change in how we address pain."

"The question of the reliability of self-report always seems to come up," I say. "Is that something Pain BC, or the Task Force, is concerned about?"

"No," Maria says bluntly. "And that's part of the paradigm shift."

She explains that the Task Force receives input from twenty-four of the most preeminent experts in the pain field and, among them, the reliability of self-report is never debated. And that's because the consensus is that asking people to prove their pain goes against even the most basic bottom-line approach. If you want people to recover, and you want to diminish costs, you don't set up a system where people must continually prove pain or disability in order to get benefits. You simply provide the support necessary so that they *can* get better.

"With this approach, ICBC is already seeing a reduction of costs, and we'll get more financial data in the years to come," Maria says. "But the real question, I think, is what does this very significant paradigmatic shift mean for health outcomes? Do outcomes improve when people no longer feel surveyed and suspected? Will the shift from acute pain to ongoing chronic pain be lessened under this new kind of system? Moving forward, that's the research I'm really interested in."

"I'm with you," I say, "but I've been challenged a few times on this topic by friends wondering how the fakers and malingers will be weeded out."

"When people say that kind of thing to me," Maria says, "I always ask, where are they getting their data? What are the numbers regarding the percentage of people scamming the system for secondary gains? Numbers we do know are that chronic pain impacts one out of five people; that's about eight million people in Canada." We discuss how the narrative surrounding the unreliability of self-report ties back into this question of what kind of pain is given legitimacy. Pain from breaking your leg, for example, is traditionally considered legitimate. But neuroscience tells us that chronic pain is often part of an ongoing maladaptive response, which connects back to many types of trauma (things like adverse childhood experiences, social or domestic violence, harmful interactions within the health care system, systemic marginalization, or precarious housing and resource insufficiency) that all contribute to an agitated nervous system.

"And that's legitimate," Maria says. "People get hung up on this idea that self-report is only good if it describes a concrete physical injury. But is that true for anybody? Can physical pain ever be totally segregated from emotional, spiritual, psychological, or social pain? No."

LIKE HANCE CLARKE, Michael Negraeff is skeptical of a medical stance that promises to fix pain, although he acknowledges that within the doctor-patient relationship it's often a dynamic that's difficult to step away from. "People come to see you desperate for solutions, and as a physician you really want to help them. But sometimes an emphasis on 'fixing' can get in the way of the kind of whole-person healing that is required to address chronic pain. It's one of the important things I learned working with a multidisciplinary team. I remember coming into a meeting with my doctor's hat on, suggesting this medication, or that intervention, trying to fix the problem. But then the psychologist said, 'Wait a minute, what I see here is a person who has nothing to look forward to in their life.' It was an aha! moment. Because, of course, it's unlikely someone will truly get better if they feel their life lacks meaning, purpose, or connection."

Michael created his own blog space, entitled *Narratives From the Neuromatrix*, specifically to explore the intersection of these two approaches—healing and curing—and to flesh out some of the contradictions inherent in living with or treating chronic pain. We discuss how cures tend to be finite, absolute. A physician *fixes* the problem, a state of affairs that is satisfying for the physician and patient alike. The problem is, it's binary. Cures work, or they don't. Healing, by contrast, is a lifelong, nonlinear, messy proposition. It requires striving for balance in multiple areas of your life and building long-lasting (but time-consuming) partnerships between patient and doctor.

One of my favorite blog posts is titled "Consistency Is for Cattle." Michael acknowledges how the messaging around chronic pain can often feel contradictory. He writes that *don't give your pain too much attention* is one of the key pieces of advice doled out to patients. But, then again, it's also important to validate the fact that there often are *no boundaries between pain and other parts of your life.*

"I'm sort of saying 'keep pain away from parts of your life' and that you can't 'keep it away' at the same time," he explains in the post. "This is likely frustrating for some. Living a life with pain is just like living a life without pain (is there such a thing?)—there are many ways to live it successfully."

"My favorite part of the blog is where you write that we are all more than our broken parts," I tell him. "You write: *I'm always wondering where I can influence the narrative in a healing manner. The power of storytelling amazes me.*"

Michael nods. "A fellow physician once told me: 'It's what you know that cures; it's who you are that heals.' It's something I've never forgotten. There are a lot of times, as a pain physician, where no matter how much you want to, you simply can't take the pain away. And so we really have to try and help people live the most fulfilling lives as possible. Because more often than not, pain endures."

"I LIKE THE DOUBLE ENTENDRE," Si says at our next TACKLING PAIN meeting. "We endure pain but, also, pain endures. And man, does it ever endure."

"Listen to this," I say, opening my copy of David Morris's *The Culture of Pain* to the bookmarked page. "The meaning of pain," I read, "like the meaning of any complex text, always remains open to impermanent personal and social interpretations. It contains areas of darkness and mystery where firm answers may be simply unavailable. Its meaning thus must leave room not only for what we know and will come to know but also for what may remain forever unknown."

"Heavy," Simon says. "That feels true in a way that is both comforting and depressing."

"Ah, the contradictions of pain."

"Right?" he says. "We've been at this TACKLING PAIN project for almost a year but... all the contradictions? All the uncertainty? It doesn't get easier with time."

"I believe the phrase you used at the outset was, 'It's fucking exhausting.'"

Simon nods. "Our metaphors may have changed over the year. But, sadly, that's still pretty much the same."

# 20

# Another Anniversary

JULY 22, 2019.

A few days later we are up past our bedtime waiting for our friend Avi Lewis to visit. The day was scorching hot, but the heat has eased by the time he knocks on our door holding an acoustic guitar and a bottle of bourbon. We've reached a point in our life where almost nothing, or no one, can alter our evening routines, but Avi is the exception.

As a journalist and filmmaker, Avi is super-busy, and we're lucky if we manage a visit once or twice a year. Especially in the last couple of years, when Avi, along with Naomi Klein—his wife and partner-in-activism—has been writing and promoting The Leap Manifesto, an urgent call to take bold steps to prevent further catastrophic global warming. Fueled by a vision of a country powered entirely by renewable energy, their action plan weaves together issues of climate justice, rights of workers, and gender, racial, and income equality.

It's been three years since the death of David Bowie—an artist Avi interviewed several times in the 1990s—and we've been trying to get together ever since to raise a toast and sing loud and slightly off-key versions of some of our favorite songs. We're always thrilled to see Avi, but especially so if it involves a sing-along.

Before we start singing, he fills us in on his latest project, a short film collaboration with the artist Molly Crabapple. Avi co-wrote the film's narration with Alexandria Ocasio-Cortez, a rising star in American politics, as a kind of thought experiment: What might the world look like if we put the concept of care—for the planet, and for one another—at the very center of our personal, public, and political lives?

Our conversation veers into a discussion of the value gap in our culture between *curing* and *caring* as it relates to both chronic pain and climate justice, and Simon briefly outlines our TACKLING PAIN project.

"I've had to continually confront my own desire for a quick fix, my own sense of entitlement to be 'cured' and to have science solve this problem for me," Simon says. "I'm finally starting to understand that healing can occur even in the absence of a cure. But healing? It's messy and time-consuming. A lot of freaking work with absolutely no guarantee of success."

"And as a society we don't value that kind of work, not really. In fact, we actively devalue it," Avi says. "Check this out." He pulls out his phone and reads out statistics from the Oxfam website:

> Women and girls undertake more than three-quarters of unpaid care work in the world and make up two-thirds of the paid care workforce. They carry out 12.5 billion hours of unpaid care work every day. When valued at minimum wage this would represent a contribution to the global economy of at least $10.8 trillion a year, more than three times the size of the global tech industry.

"That's... gross," I say. Simon likes to joke that I've put in enough caregiving hours over the last decade to qualify as an *un*registered nurse. Personally, I resist applying the word *caregiver* to myself, preferring to categorize our relationship with more marital equanimity: we care for each other. That's the way it's always been. Still, the aftermath of brain and spinal cord injuries comes with a few undeniable facts. I have had to assume a lopsided burden of physical caregiving duties, a state that will only become more challenging as we both age. Time spent caregiving has placed restrictions on my work life, and there are long-term financial consequences related to this. But consistent care and support at home has meant on several occasions that Simon has not had to be hospitalized, as many others would have in different circumstances.

"The argument is always that better care will require more money," I say. "But short-term 'cures' that don't address the complexity of pain, or the root causes, mean that often the problem only gets bigger. Throw in substance-use disorders and you have a social problem that comes at an enormous emotional and financial cost. Everyone pays: individuals, families, medical systems, society as a whole. There's no way investing in educational and care-based solutions alongside traditional medical approaches is more costly. It just requires a readjustment of our values. More preemptive medicine instead of always doing damage control."

"You mean, build a roadside guardrail," Simon says. "Instead of parking a caravan of ambulances at the bottom of the cliff."

"Exactly." Simon is invoking an image used by Harvard Medical School professor Jeffrey Rediger to describe America's current health care system. It's become a shorthand in our house for situations where investing in long-term and sustainable preventative measures is always preferable—and more cost-efficient—than waiting for a predictable disaster to occur.

"Denmark's a good practical example," Avi says. "They have more extensive universal health care services, but they spend less, per capita, than we do on health care costs."

We continue to discuss how some of the most challenging questions around the global burden of chronic pain *and* climate justice center on this notion of care. How, in societies where the feminine-associated concepts of care and cooperation are devalued and exploited, are we all holding up? What is lost when ruggedly individualized notions of health and continual self-improvement (available, really, only to those with enough cash to buy into an ever-expanding self-care industry) replace a focus on collective, communal health? And what is the cumulative cost of an unsustainable and extractive world cosmology that views our earth, and the vast array of life it sustains, as somehow separate and distinct from our vulnerable and mortal human bodies, instead of recognizing that the health of every living entity is intimately connected to the health of our planet as a whole?

"If the epidemic of chronic pain is any barometer," I say, "we—at least one in five of us—are not holding up all that well. We're in pain. We're suffering."

"It's hard, right?" Avi says. "Fighting for climate justice requires us to consider, or at least attempt to consider, at all times, all the intersecting systems: the biological, the ecological, the historical, the economic, the social, the spiritual, the political."

"Chronic pain too," I say.

"And putting care at the forefront of that fight requires that we recognize our very human interdependency."

"To interdependency," Si says, raising his bourbon glass, ice cubes clinking.

"And to Bowie," Avi says.

"We'll start with 'Five Years'?" Si strums the opening chords.

"Right," Avi says. "Then let's do 'Soul Love.'"

"I'M A LITTLE TIPSY," Simon says from the bed as I pull on my nightshirt.

"Are you okay?"

"Yeah. Just—can you fill my water glass? I'll need to hydrate."

I head to the kitchen, noticing the flashing red light indicating an unplayed message on our phone.

"Hey," I say, placing the water glass on Si's bedside table. "Your mom left a message earlier today to say she was thinking about us. Today is the twenty-second—the eleventh anniversary of your accident and the first anniversary of our TACKLING PAIN project."

"Whoa," Si says. "I totally forgot."

"Right? Me too. I know we haven't seen a huge reduction of your pain. But forgetting this date? That weirdly seems like a marker of success."

"Yeah," Si says. "And it's fitting that tonight was so much fun." It's almost 2:30, and Avi left about a half hour ago after a late, loud night. We ran through all the hits—including an extra-dramatic version of "Ziggy Stardust"—and Avi regaled us with his up-close-and-personal moments with the iconic David Bowie. "Tonight was the kind of medicine I've been needing for a long time."

I crawl into bed, smiling, and not just because I too am a little tipsy. I love this idea of a rare moment with Avi, sharing songs and stories, as being a kind of medicine. "Imagine if our not-so-mythic multidisciplinary pain clinic had a section for non-medical prescriptions."

"I like it. A musician could prescribe songs; a writer, poems."

For the next few minutes we engage in a whimsical brainstorm. It begins with a camping prescription: sit by an open fire near a lake and eat canned beans while watching the stars come out. Next a philosophy prescription: read Bertrand Russell on why love is wise and hatred foolish, or Oliver Sacks's musings on the topic of gratitude. Then an entirely predictable puppy prescription, which is really a prescription for warm-bodied play and boundless but clumsy devotion. I suggest a travel prescription—go someplace you've never been before—which Simon vetoes for a learning-a-new-instrument prescription.

"What would be your new instrument?" I ask.

"Trumpet, definitely."

"How about a dance party prescription?" I say.

"Always a good option."

"And a social activism prescription?"

"Yeah. Hmm," Simon says. "Avi's political passion is... inspiring. It makes me realize that all my focus is split between pain and performing. It's all very self-involved. I really do need a social activism prescription."

"What would you do?"

"I'm not sure. I'll have to think about it."

Whimsy spent, we return more seriously to imagining what would happen if the concept of care was placed at the very center of our communal life. Multidisciplinary pain clinics might then be embedded in much larger community care, or wellness, centers. Instead of post-secondary education in return for military service, we would perhaps see an exchange of education for care service, offering young people real-world experience at initiatives designed to care, in a sustainable way, for our environment, for our public spaces, for our young, for our elders, for the marginalized and vulnerable in our communities. Along with birth or death doulas, we might see an increase in chronic pain or chronic illness doulas, so that people might be supported not only in navigating their medical appointments but also in finding empowerment in other areas of their life. A person-in-pain might be able, with the necessary support, to be involved in cultivating community gardens, recycling programs, tool-or-time share-shed initiatives, or education and awareness programs designed to combat racial or gender injustice.

"It's really important to have the opportunity to be a caregiver too," Simon says. "Not, you know, just a terminal care receiver." He takes a long sip of water, then turns to face me, and busts out a deep belly laugh. "Oh, Stanley. I can see the thoughts racing across your face."

"One thing—"

"Enough," he says. "It's three o'clock. I'm done talking."

"But—"

"Nope, no buts. Happy anniversary." He switches off his light. "Peace out, girlfriend."

IT'S A SLOW START to the day the following morning. Over breakfast, to commemorate our first TACKLING PAIN anniversary, we compile a list:

IMPORTANT THINGS WE HAVE HAD TO LEARN; LEARN AGAIN; AND WILL LIKELY HAVE TO LEARN ALL OVER IN THE FUTURE.

1) ADDRESS STRESS.

Be rigorous in identifying and confronting the factors that generate stress. Understand

—that stressful factors belong to multiple domains: the biological, the psychological, and the social.

—that habitual thought patterns might be amplifying or even creating unnecessary stress.

—that habitual movement patterns, too, might be amplifying or even creating stress in your body.

Acknowledge that these two things—thought and movement—are intrinsically interconnected. Accept that ignoring any kind of stress will only make it worse. Take concrete action to address and control what you can while accepting that some things will always be out of your control. Resist the sometimes insistent urge to catastrophize possible future events.

2) FOCUS ON THE PROCESS, NOT THE GOAL.

Everyone's process will be unique and should play to individual strengths and reflect individual values. Understand that making change is often slow. It is a long-term commitment that requires honesty and awareness. Don't expect instantaneous results. Give yourself permission to routinely experiment with being the tortoise, not the hare. Trust in your process and try, as much as possible, to find pleasure in the ride.

3) WHEN ALL ELSE FAILS: BREATHE. JUST BREATHE.
Breathing is an automatic function. But it's *also* a movement powered by the strong contraction and release of the diaphragm, and with attention and practice this muscular action can be strengthened and improved. The first and last act of any living creature, breathing is the most fundamental way in which we nourish and cleanse our bodies. Learning how to breathe more capaciously is almost always possible. Better breathing = better mental and physical health.

4) CHOOSE GRATITUDE.
It's a word that gets used a lot these days, but it is, ultimately, what determines the texture of our daily life. Make the choice to let your thankfulness for what you have and who you are outweigh your grief and anger for the absence of the things you've lost along the way—

"But, also," I say, interrupting our list-making, "leave a little room for—what did you call it?—*baditude?* When things are really tough, I know I default to focusing on my gratitudes—and I *am* grateful for so much, for you, for Eli, for the life we share, along with a lot of other things, like fresh peaches and early morning swims and the way Chico plows his head into my knee when he wants an ear scratch—but sometimes a little kick of anger is necessary too. To make change."

"Right," Simon says. He amends the title to read *Choose gratitude (with a little latitude for baditude)* before we move on to number—

5) SEEK CONNECTIONS.
Between your moving and thinking body. Between your internal and external world. Between yourself and others.

It's these connections that help us find the strength and resilience to . . .

6) EMBRACE THE MYSTERY.

Aging, illness, and chronic pain are not just medical problems. They are all aspects that more rightly belong to the vast, trembling, achingly beautiful, and ultimately mysterious realm of human mortality. Embracing this mystery means allowing for the possibility of uncertainty and contradiction—

"Or maybe," Si interjects, "embracing the mystery is more about deciding on a course of action, committing to it, even though you have doubts. Then, also, being open to changing course if you need to."

"That's good," I say, scribbling.

"And let's add something about all the obnoxious pain platitudes."

"Okay," I say. "What?"

"Well, you know I love good sport-isms. And focusing on some of them helped when I was in the early days of rehab. *Attitude determines altitude. Hard work beats talent when talent doesn't work hard. Experience is what happens when things don't go your way.* But I hate—*hate*—all the pain platitudes."

We make a quick list of some of the catchphrases we've run into over the past year:

· What the mind suppresses the body expresses.
· Hurt doesn't equal harm.
· Motion is lotion.
· The issue's not the tissue.
· Pain denied is pain amplified.
· No pain, no gain.
· Mind over matter.

"I mean, if a certain phrase helps someone out of a sticky situation or motivates them, then, of course, yippee. That's great," Simon says. "The problem is, every time you try and reduce the experience of living with pain into a sound bite, you'll inevitably push that 'solution' into contradiction or error. You can't be absolutist."

I nod. He's right. There is, for example, the ridiculousness of the phrase *mind over matter* in the context of the childhood experience of Graeme, one of Simon's key musical collaborators. Graeme was born with an exceedingly rare genetic disorder that, while resembling dwarfism, has unique and unusual characteristics, the most visible of which is an extreme hypermobility of his joints. Now thirty, he lives with what his rheumatologist says is best described as a severe state of arthritis. But Graeme also endured several invasive and extremely painful operations as a child. Once, when he was ten, he underwent a procedure, without any form of anesthetic, in a small clinic. Both his legs had been previously broken by his doctor and reset with large pins screwed through the bone above and below his knee, and in his hips; now it was time to remove these pins. "Drill?" the doctor asked ten-year old Graeme. "Or tire iron?"

Graeme, thinking that using a non-electrical tool would be less painful, chose the tire iron. "I was wrong," he told me and Simon, laughing.

When the doctor began to manually unscrew the pins, the pain was excruciating. It was deep, invasive, radiating out from inside the marrow of his bones. He began to scream. A nurse entered the room and told him to control himself and be quiet: he was frightening the children in the waiting room. When the doctors started on the second screw, Graeme lost consciousness. That experience set a pretty high pain bar. His ongoing joint pain is a defining aspect of his life, but one where a little *mind over matter* can, in small doses, be helpful. More helpful, though, is the fact that he's built a career that enables him to respect his limits and work within them. But as far as pure pain voltage? Nothing in his life has ever compared to the intensity of that procedure. "I was a respectful type of ten-year-old kid," Graeme explained. "But, boy, would my thirty-year-old self like to have a few choice words with that nurse who told me I should shut up."

"There's always a risk that a platitude will be reductive or trivializing," I say now to Simon. "Or just plain wrong."

"What was it that Sharon said to you?" Simon asks, referring to a friend of ours newly recovering from a surgery to remove half her sigmoid colon. A quintessentially non-catastrophizing type of personality, Sharon had repeatedly told me prior to this invasive surgery that it was a no-fret situation and, in the end, she was right: both the procedure and her recovery were, by all objective measures, a success. Still, at seventy-five, Sharon's recovery included a fair share of up-and-down days and worrisome—and painful—moments as her digestive system acclimated to eating again. She navigated those difficult days by rigorously tuning in to the messages of her body.

"She said her philosophy about pain was that 'sometimes it is just noise, and sometimes it is useful information, and it matters to distinguish,'" I say. "And that's the central dilemma, right? In so many situations it's tough to distinguish. Is this pain noise? Or is it critical info necessary for my ongoing survival? It's hard to provide clear guidance with a sound bite," I say. "What's the platitude you like the least?"

"Easy," he says. "*Pain is inevitable, suffering isn't.*"

"Okay. Explain."

"Well, it's true, mostly. It's common sense. You can always make a bad situation worse. You can focus on feeling sorry for yourself, or feeling angry, or fearful, or blaming someone for what's happening. All of that is going to increase your suffering. When I can keep a check on those things, life is better. But saying suffering isn't inevitable? That's glib, arrogant, patronizing. And, also, wrong. Pain has an impact. And sometimes, especially when I can't see an end in sight, I get weary. I get sad. Sometimes I suffer. Sometimes I see *you* suffering, and that makes me suffer too. It's too facile to say that by speaking truth to that lived experience, I'm somehow shaping it. The essential kernel of truth becomes diminished—and I become resistant to it—when all that complexity is reduced into a snappy sound bite. One that doesn't recognize the difficulty we all face when having to hold two or more opposing ideas as potentially true. Suffering isn't inevitable; suffering, in life, is inevitable. Both statements deserve respect."

"Consistency," I say, quoting Michael Negraeff, "is for cattle."

"Right? And maybe it's *more* true to say that often we need to move through a necessary phase of suffering for true healing to occur, in the same way that sometimes you need to move through a certain amount of pain before you get better. It's the getting stuck—in suffering or in pain—that's the problem, not the suffering or the pain itself."

"Smart," I say.

"I'm trying," he says. "What about you? Do you have any 'aha!' thoughts after our year?"

"Well, the people I talked to who all manage what appears to be an unmanageable amount of pain—and I put you on that list—all had a few things in common. Mostly, they still had a sense of humor *and* they refused to privilege their pain over the pain of others."

"How do you mean?"

"Well, like you. You always talk about how impossible it is to fully know another person's pain."

"Yeah, I guess. Everyone's got their own boulder to push up that hill," Si says, then points at our busy brainstorm sheet. "Are you going to type this out?"

"Silly question. Of course I am."

"Would you print a copy? On tough days it would help to have it on hand. A quick cheat sheet to remind me to get my head right—even if my body's not behaving."

"Sure," I say.

"You know, a large part of the reason this past year has been good is that it's not only our metaphors or our language that has changed. It's the moment-by-moment experience of pain that's shifted. You've helped me to get curious. Pain sucks, but... it's also become a little interesting. Something to think about, something to question—and not just something to constantly react to."

"Cool," I say. "That's really cool."

# 21

# Enduring Pain

SECRET PLACES

Lovers find secret places
Inside this violent world
Where they make transactions
With beauty.

Reason says, Nonsense.
I have walked and measured the walls here.
There are no places like that.

Love says, There are.

RUMI

JANUARY 12, 2020.

In my dream, Simon and I are in our old living room in the house we lived in before his accident. Simon is standing. Beyond the curve of his broad shoulder is the living room window. Outside it's summer. The hydrangea is bursting with fat blooms, a soft shade of lavender. Under a low-hanging bough lurks an ugly turkey vulture. Its neck is long and serpentine, its feathers glossy black. "Look," I say, interrupting Simon mid-sentence. "There's a turkey vulture in the yard."

In the dreamscape, Simon turns to look out the window.

Beside me, in bed, he starts to scream. He grabs at the bedsheets, pulling himself upright, dragging us both out of sleep.

For a moment, it's as if the turkey vulture is there, its inky feathers part of the darkness, then I blink and the bird is gone and I'm awake.

Simon's cries escalate as he leans forward. He is possessed. He grabs the comforter, leaning over his legs. If he could, he would climb out of his body. I reach my hands to his cranium and sacrum, placing my fingers with a soft but solid touch.

"Fifty-seven times thirteen," I say.

There is a pause. He inhales. "Seven hundred and..." he exhales. "Seven hundred and forty-one. Thank you. Dit Dat?"

"Of course." He hands me a bottle of Dit Dat Jiao, our preferred topical pain remedy, made by our friend and local herbalist Mary Boulding. During the day, we always use the full name, overemphasizing the last word—Dit Dat *Jiaaaaoow*—but at night, when every bit of energy is economized, it's just Dit Dat. I sprinkle it over the lower half of his back, careful not to splash it on the sheets. It stains terribly.

"Thanks," he says again and then starts coughing, a violent hacking that sets off another back spasm.

"Okay?" I ask when it finally passes.

"Yeah," he says, lying back down. "I'm okay."

I press play on the iPad and as the low, slow frequencies of Tibetan singing bowls reverberate, Simon's breath slows and he softens into sleep beside me.

Outside, the weather is the exact opposite of my balmy dreamscape. The rain clatters in the eaves and the wind, unusually turbulent, has transformed the distant humming pulse of the sea into a lawless bluster and crash. It's perfect weather for pulling the duvet covers over your head and sleeping long and late.

But now I'm stubbornly awake, caught in reliving an incident from a week ago. Simon was finishing up a gig, a Sunday afternoon jam at a golf club, when an unexpected snow squall hit. We packed up quickly and he drove us through whiteout conditions, our wheelchair-accessible van sliding through the sharp turns, steep inclines, and precipitous descents on the narrow highway home—a forty-minute trip that took easily twice that long. For a moment at the outset of that white-knuckle drive, my worrying mind ran ahead with a series of fearful what-ifs. What if the van slides into a ditch? How would Simon get out of the van? We wouldn't be able to deploy the wheelchair ramp so he could wheel out and transferring out the door of his elevated driver's seat into his wheelchair would be impossible—too high, too difficult, and I wasn't strong enough to lift him out. And, even if he could get out of the van, how would we get the wheelchair home over hilly, snow-covered roads? I could call our friends Joe and Amy, both strong and resourceful in an emergency, but even with the extra manpower I'm not sure we could solve those issues. Would I have to call 911? Get firefighters to come? In a snowstorm? My thoughts spiraled out. Then I recalled some of the incidental life lessons that had been so thoroughly underscored during our TACKLING PAIN project. *Stop catastrophizing. Focus on the present moment. Trust yourself to deal with an issue when, or if, you have to.* All things that are easy to say but, especially in a potential crisis, surprisingly difficult to do. I shushed the chattering voices in my head, leaned forward, and focused on helping Simon see the road ahead.

When we made it home, Simon confessed to navigating the exact same thought process.

"Before your accident, neither of us would have sweated it," I said. "If the road got too bad, we would have parked the van and walked home."

"Yeah," Si shrugged. "It might have taken half the night, but it would have been an adventure."

I find myself indulging in a deep moment of... what? Self-pity? Anger? Frustration? It is, really, a complicated mix of all three. I hate our constant state of vulnerability. I hate how things that used to be easy are now difficult, and things that were difficult often feel impossible. I hate the fact that I'm not big and strong and competent enough to better minimize that sense of vulnerability for Simon. If our positions were reversed and I was the one in the wheelchair, the problems posed by the snowstorm wouldn't have been so dire. Simon would have simply lifted me out of the van, carrying me home in his arms, if he had to. Chronic pain, as we've spent the last decade learning and relearning, results when there is an abundance of perceived threat—either biological, psychological, or environmental—and an absence of stability. How much, I wonder, does my inability to provide a sense of physical safety for Simon contribute to his chronic pain?

But there's another life lesson that our year of TACKLING PAIN has underscored: forgiveness and self-compassion are important. We are, I remind myself now, trying our best. And, fuck it, if there are days—and there are many—when we aren't at our best, well, that's okay too.

We gave up counting our TACKLING PAIN days after the first anniversary, but nothing has stopped. Si's maintained his journaling, his Dreampad time, and his meditation. We do the qigong movement together a few times a week. He's added short wheels down our street to the frog pond, gradually rebuilding some of his strength. Over the summer he committed to a daily ten minutes of weeding the vegetable gardens. And, taking his own social activism prescription seriously, he has become involved in the Disability Foundation: now, along with being a longtime contributing member of the Vancouver Adapted Music Society, Simon volunteers on the board of directors for the Disabled Independent Gardeners Association, helping to promote gardening opportunities for people in the disability community.

Less successful have been Simon's attempts to lower his hydromorphone use. Small gains are made, but with any kind of change, they're quickly lost. Recently there was a malfunction in the seat cushion of his wheelchair, and that, along with his wicked cough and low-grade fever, caused a massive spike in pain. After a year of slowly reducing his opioid intake, he's back to the same dosage he was on for the last ten years.

So the project continues.

But, I am realizing, continuing to use the word *project* is just another way to trick myself into thinking that the hard work of confronting the pain will one day be over. As if sometime soon we'll simply be able to halt our unscientific experiment and get back to real life. But this *is* our life and this is the work ahead.

The difficulty, I tell myself, is that the more you look at the problem of pain, the bigger it gets. If pain was a stone dropped into the waters of the world, it would create infinitely expanding ripples. It is unending. Trying to get a glimpse of the whole is about as easy as holding a scoop of that water in your hand.

It's a tough realization, because what Si and I both want—what anyone wants, really—is for our project to have a happy ending.

It's not that the *unending* I foresee now is necessarily unhappy, exactly. It's just also messy, confusing, unfinished. Difficult. Real, I guess.

Ten percent. By Simon's current calculation, his pain, because of our year-plus interventions, is approximately ten percent better—a modest number, but, still, it's a start. A place to build from. The insight, he says, that has resonated most deeply for him was something pain activist Joletta Belton said: *I needed to stop focusing on changing the pain and start focusing on changing my life.*

That piece of wisdom, so generously given, helped Simon make a big life decision. He's chosen not to book any gigs with his band for at least a year, as he normally would after releasing an album. It's too much pressure right now. Instead, he's playing two low-key Sunday afternoon jams a month. They're open jams, so as the afternoon unfolds, the house band (with Simon on guitar) is joined by scores of jammers, ranging from kickass professionals to aspiring musicians. It's an inclusive environment that encourages musical risk taking, and the house band has to be agile as it improvises behind the wide range of talent. It's fun. The band plays familiar music, songs that people love, and everyone dances and sings along.

"Hopefully it won't be forever," Simon said when he made the decision to limit Farm Team gigs. "But it's a way to maintain my skills as a playing musician without so much stress. I need to redefine my relationship to playing live again." It's a compromise, but it allows for the flexibility Simon needs to keep working.

As we did in the aftermath of his accident, we're once again reconciling ourselves to the fact that healing is a lifelong process, one that sometimes imposes difficult-to-accept limitations.

"I don't think I'm ever going to fully grow out of hoping that science will solve this for me. A pill, or a procedure. A phone call out of the blue from Dr. Heran with compelling new data for an improved ablation technique," Simon said recently, over a dinnertime TACKLING PAIN conversation. "It might sound foolish, but I still want to believe in that miracle."

"You *want* to *believe*," I said. "Is that the same thing as *wanting* to *believe* that one day a shark will stop attacking you? It's still a pretty big leap of faith."

"Well, what is faith," Si said, "if not a kind of soulful hope that persists, even in the absence of guaranteed answers or outcomes?"

"Pain, my love, is turning you into a philosopher."

He grinned. "Well. Along with that hope, I also worry that the chaos of two summers ago could return at any time."

"It could," I said. "Not to be a bummer, but it likely will. That's life, right?"

"Maybe after this last year, we'll have a few more resources to help us move through the chaos."

This, I realize now as I listen to Simon's ragged snores, might be as close to a happy ending as we will get: there are no quick fixes, no easy answers, just a commitment to each other, the kind of for-better-or-for-worse promise that builds a marriage into an ever-sturdier structure, a tempered, tested, and forgiving love that shelters us in a place of relative safety and pleasure, no matter what loss, heartache, or pain might come our way. Loving each other, ourselves, our work, and the earth we live on is our best, most powerful, antidote to life's inevitable phases of chaos, grief, and suffering.

It's still too early to rise, but a return to sleep seems increasingly unlikely. Morning is coming. A poet friend refers to this dusky liminal space between night and day as *wolflight,* a word I love. Beside me, Simon's breath echoes the wet turbulence of the wind, rain, and sea. Recently several news stories have detailed a precipitous rise in cases of a mysterious respiratory infection. It's like SARS, maybe. One news story suggested it spread from bats to humans; another suggested a pangolin-to-human transmission. Neither Simon nor I had ever heard of a pangolin, and when we looked it up online we were delighted with both its absurdly scaly anteater body and the lovely skip of syllables in its name. Now we refer to Simon's increasingly soupy chest infection as the *pangolin flu.* It isn't, of course. The news reports insist that all the cases of this mysterious virus are still contained within Chinese borders.

"Stan?" Simon says, and then starts coughing. Once again, he struggles to sit up in bed. This chest infection has, over the last twenty-four hours, turned nasty.

"Yeah?"

"Am I keeping you awake? I'm sorry I keep coughing."

"No, I can't sleep. It's not your fault. Do you think your cough is worse?"

"It is. It almost feels like I'm drowning. If it gets worse, it might mean a trip to the ER."

"Okay." Outside, the wind chimes clatter and the rain ricochets off the window. Dawn has finally arrived: wet and gray, loud and unruly. "How about we make it a full-on sick day? Nothing productive allowed. Just cozy time: movies, soup, and ginger tea. What do you think?"

"Perfect," Si says.

# 22

# The Thing With Feathers

MARCH 2020.

Chaos, as it turns out, is not so far away.

The week of March ninth is memorable. Monday, we are still making plans. Midweek, the world has gone sideways. Everything is canceled. By Friday the whole world has changed, and around the globe people struggle to understand life's rapidly transforming rules of engagement. My friend Jane sends out an email: *Monday*, she writes, *was a simpler time.*

In the end, Si's winter cough resolved quickly with no need for a visit to the doctor. We've been consoling ourselves with the speculation that perhaps it was indeed an advance Covid-19 infection, and now Si is one of the few who has some immunities. We're aware that even by magical-thinking standards, this is a weak, grasping narrative. But ever since we learned that along with his health issues, one of Si's medications places him at an increased risk of contracting the rapidly spreading virus, he has felt anxious. After more than a year of parsing out the relationship between the threat of danger and pain, we've decided it's critical to, as Simon says, keep it cozy. *Be easy, bruv.*

Some days minimizing anxiety is easier said than done. All over the world threat levels skyrocket. The invisible menace of an airborne virus combined with the economic and social peril that accompanies the isolation of quarantine fuels a nuclear-level fire at the core of global pain.

And then other days, despite this looming threat, it's not so hard at all. Other days, life insists on itself. The tenacity of spring flowers is an excellent antidote to anxiety. We have the luxury of time to sit together on the front porch and watch the hummingbirds zooming in and out of the frilly azalea blooms. All around us small dramas unfold. A territorial debate rages between the crows that live in the tall cedar, discussions ranging from animated to livid. Occasionally violence breaks out. And an adolescent deer, unafraid of Chico, has taken to jumping the fence into our yard. After a few failed attempts at chasing the bold fellow, Chico decides his best strategy is distraction. So, while the deer decimates the plum tree and rose bushes in the back yard, then lies down to nap in the dry grass, Chico busies himself in the front yard, aggressively barking at a harmless squirrel.

"Best reality show ever," Si says.

A sticky yellow layer of pollen covers the windshield of my car, and my slightly swollen glands and drippy nose are entirely predictable. Still. Three days ago, there was that woman in the health food store who was stridently refusing to wear a mask. I realize that I am going to have to go through a period of worry after every foray to get groceries. Each outside contact now brings the fear that I might carry the virus home to Simon. And it's hard not to take it personally when someone adopts an ideological stance against current public health measures—like masking up—that are meant to reduce harm and protect the vulnerable. Even at the most prosperous and optimistic of times, there is a divide between the perspectives of those who must directly contend with life's fragility and those who don't; now, as polarizing rhetoric infects social media, that divide seems likely, at least for a little while, to turn into an unbridgeable chasm.

*This is going to get much worse before there is any chance that it will get better.* Those were the trauma doctor's words to me in the immediate aftermath of Simon's accident. *Worse than this?* I had thought. *Impossible.* I find myself remembering those words on a daily basis.

"In a way, we've spent the last decade preparing for this moment," Simon says. We're out on the front porch eating a late dinner. What he says is true. We already know what it means to have to radically slow down. We've had a long time to grapple with the fact that science doesn't always have all the answers and when the answers do come, they might not be entirely risk-free. Sometimes the choices available aren't ideal. You must decide for yourself what the least worst choice will be and try to make the best of it. Is the benefit worth the risk?

"It's maybe a terrible thing to admit," Simon says, swallowing a last bit of taco and wiping cilantro sauce from his fingers, "but along with the worry I'm experiencing a huge amount of relief. Unqualified. There have been so many times since my accident that I've been sidelined with health issues, so many gigs I've had to turn down or cancel. I hate being left out of things. But now I get a break, and the rest of the world is on break with me. I'm not the only guy missing out."

"It's strange, that combination of worry and relief," I agree, gathering up our dinner plates. The sky is dark purple now and the angular outlines of bats pitch in and out of the shadowy limbs of the cedar trees. "Worry for the world at large but, simultaneously, thankful for this slowed-down time. That breathless sense of always running late, or of drowning in a to-do list I never ever get on top of, is fading."

"Aside from rehab, it's the first time in my adult life that I don't have a gig on the horizon," Simon says as he rolls into the kitchen.

"True."

"If I were to quit hydromorphone, now would be the time to do it."

"Yeah," I say. "It would." Over the spring, Simon had once again succeeded in reducing his hydromorphone use, but he stalled out at about ten milligrams in a twenty-four-hour period and couldn't seem to get it lower. I want to discuss this further, but fearful that I won't be able to hide my sudden spark of excitement, I clam up.

The following morning, Simon wakes at dawn. "There's been music playing in my mind all night. A new song. It won't let me sleep. I have to get it down before I lose it," he says, transferring into his wheelchair and leaving me, unusually, lingering alone in bed. "It's about kicking hydromorphone," he adds, as he wheels out of the room.

Snuggled into our summer sheets, I listen as Simon goes straight to his guitar and begins to play. *You can tell me once, you can tell me twice,* he sings. *Just coz you say it three times, don't make it good advice.* Verses spill out of him as if he's spent a week memorizing them, but it's when he reaches the chorus that I pay close attention. *You think you got the best of me,* he growls. *But that's the last of me you'll get.*

*Oh, there it is,* I think, happy and surprisingly unsurprised. *He's made up his mind to quit.*

The next three days pass in a quasi-spatial haze. Without his regular doses of hydromorphone, Si is a little discombobulated. He reports that his left arm is unusually achy and his sleeps are somewhat erratic. But he doesn't get nauseous, and there are no long stretches of insomnia, and, most amazingly, no significant overall increase in pain. The pain is there, of course, neuropathic stabs and surges, same as always, but it hasn't gone berserk. By the third morning Simon's digestion is not so sluggish, and (though it could be my imagination) I'm certain he's shed some of his usual gray pallor. There's a little of his old rosy cheek visible now.

For so long, quitting hydromorphone was an overwhelming proposition. But the withdrawal? It hasn't been so excruciating. Now, by the fourth day, things are relatively stable. Simon has a busy day attending an online board meeting for the Disability Foundation and a group planning session for a new radio podcast project. He demos the new blues song and teaches two guitar lessons over Zoom. All to say, he's easily making it through a relatively normal day.

Wow.

After five days, he explains that it feels as if he is waking from an extended dream state. "The fog is dissipating," he says. "I'm more clear-headed."

The sixth night he is restless, but the next morning he rises earlier than usual. As Chico and I prepare to head out for a morning walk, Si asks if he can come.

It's nine o'clock in the morning. He hasn't voluntarily been out of the house that early in a very long time.

We drive to the Hidden Grove forest. "Time to take a forest bath," I say, as he rolls into a stand of towering old-growth trees.

When we get home, he plays guitar for over an hour.

Then he goes for a swim.

Next he sorts the stacks of sheet music and teaching materials that had grown over the past few years like an aggressive ivy choking out all the free space in his small music studio. With the clutter sorted into an accordion file folder, the room suddenly seems twice its usual size.

Late afternoon, we go for a *second* walk, this time to the frog pond, and then we shoot hoops in the yard for almost an hour. "Sweet, Wheels McSwish," I say when Si sinks a distance shot that doesn't even graze the rim.

"It's been that kind of day, Stanley Buckets," Si says. "Kind of charmed." He catches his own rebound and fires a second shot into the center of the basket. "Today, I just can't miss."

In bed, later in the evening, he opens his left arm so I can snuggle into the notch under his collarbone. "You know, quitting hydromorphone was a really difficult decision," he says. "But now? It's strangely anticlimactic."

"Yeah?"

"It's a pretty good feeling."

"Yeah."

COVID WAS NEVER MEANT to be a part of our TACKLING PAIN project, a curveball neither of us could have anticipated. But in a story dedicated to the topic of persistent pain, and the related factors of stress and uncertainty, it can't be ignored. As the pandemic months passed we bore witness to the ways in which marginalized communities were disproportionately impacted, just as they are with chronic pain, both vivid examples of the ways our physical bodies are changeable landscapes, shaped not only by biological forces but by social and political ones as well.

There is some irony in the fact that the limits imposed by the pandemic increased Simon's overall sense of health and well-being, the additional time and space assisting him to make, and follow through on, the difficult decision to quit taking opioids. Sadly, his is not a typical story. For many people suffering from persistent pain, lockdown meant a disruption of necessary in-person appointments. The extra strain on already overtaxed medical systems resulted in further barriers for the treatment of a condition that's still routinely misunderstood and poorly managed.

In July 2020, our province had to recognize that it was in the midst of not one but two catastrophic public health crises: Covid *and* death by overdose. More people in British Columbia died of overdose in May and June of 2020 than in any other month since the onset of the overdose crisis in 2016. At that time, the overall rate of overdose deaths in the province was 20 people per 100,000 residents. By 2021, that number had more than doubled, to 41 people per 100,000.

"Since 2016 overdose deaths in B.C. have had a few things in common," I say to Simon, reading to him from a recent Pain BC newsletter. "They were mostly male, many worked in construction or related industries, and at least half were living with pain."

"In a parallel universe that could be me," Simon says.

"Yep. I'm glad it isn't."

The efforts of our TACKLING PAIN project didn't result in a significant reduction in Simon's overall pain—just small, often barely discernable, improvements. But now, reading the heartbreaking statistics of drug deaths, I wonder: Was Simon empowered to make the decision to quit opioids in part because of all the work he put in over that year? It would be impossible to prove, but it also seems reasonable to believe.

WE SPEND A LOT OF TIME on our sunny front porch. Chico keeps watch from the shady, riotous patch of vinca underneath the mountain ash tree as Simon bends the strings of his Santa Cruz guitar and serenades the trees, his song giving voice to tumultuous emotion the way that only music can.

The father of my closest childhood friend died last week. His name was Bruce, and his wife of fifty-seven years, Sophie, also suffering from Covid, was not able to be with him. Veronica, his daughter, spent hours on the phone late into his last night, long past the time he could make any response, listening to his troubled breath. She read aloud from Oliver Sacks's book *Gratitude.* "I wasn't able to be there," she told me the following morning. "But at least I was able to say everything that I wanted him to hear: that he was unique in the world; that he was loved. That he will be remembered."

A death like that, with loved ones separated at the moment they most want and need to be together, is a tragedy, a very personal tragedy but one writ large across the globe. The ancient Greeks understood tragedy as an art form that has the capacity to pull away the shimmering curtain between life and death, unveiling the truth that there are forces within our world that we cannot contain or defeat, and serving to remind humanity that we are not above, or beyond, or outside the natural world. All our fates are interconnected. We grow and thrive and we sicken and suffer because we are mortal: adaptable, creative, vulnerable, limited physical beings.

Our TACKLING PAIN project has taught us that pain, like a brilliant Greek tragedy, asks us to pay attention to difficult things. To not always numb, deny, or distract when we are uncomfortable. Pain asks questions of us that are challenging, maybe even impossible, to answer definitively. But perhaps the point isn't that we always know the answers. Perhaps, instead, we must strive to ask better and better questions. The buried hope at the heart of tragedy is that by not turning away from suffering, or its inevitable progression towards death, we may approach something essential that allows us a brief glimpse of the great mysteries that reverberate beyond the edges of our everyday awareness.

"A brief glimpse, okay," Simon says. "But sometimes enough is enough. You can only stare into that abyss for so long. Sometimes you have to whistle past that graveyard." We're both looking forward to what a post–TACKLING PAIN project, post-pandemic world will bring. And life, thankfully, is shifting back toward normal. Simon is in the process of booking bands for an outdoor summer music series at our local beachside park. In a few months' time, there will be dancing and beer gardens and ocean swims with friends I haven't seen in months. "And Chico can come," Si says. "He'll love it."

"Sounds—"

"Fun! Right? Sometimes you need a little fun to restore your hope for humanity."

"Emily Dickinson," I say, "believed that hope is the thing with feathers."

"Nice. I like that definition best." Simon picks up the Santa Cruz. "Want to play a song?"

"Sure," I say.

"'Hard Times'?" he asks. Written by Gillian Welch and David Rawlings and recorded on the album *The Harrow & the Harvest*, it's easily our household's most played tune of the last few years.

"Sure," I say, as he strums the opening chords.

*Hard times,* we harmonize on the chorus, *ain't gonna rule my mind.* It's a refrain that has a rumbling resonance. Together, we raise our voices, fearlessly, if a little out of tune, each time repeating the chorus with renewed intent and resolution. It is a promise we make to one another:

*Hard times... ain't gonna rule my mind... no more.*

# Acknowledgments

SPECIAL THANKS

OVER THE COURSE OF MY RESEARCH I spoke with several people who, like Simon, had searched both inside and outside of the medical system to find practical pain solutions and strategies. I owe them immense gratitude for their time, openness, and honesty.

One of Simon's all-time favorite musical collaborators, **Graeme Wyman** was born with an exceedingly rare genetic disorder that has resulted in a lifelong familiarity with persistent pain. As the program director for the Disability Foundation, Graeme has hands-on experience providing life-affirming opportunities to people who face a variety of accessibility challenges—he does in real life what we could only imagine happening at our mythic multidisciplinary wellness centers.

**Christa Couture** is an accomplished writer, musician, and broadcaster. She has survived cancer, first as a child and then again later in life. As a mother of two children who died before their second birthdays, she is also on intimate terms with a grief-pain that never fully recedes. She tells her own story in *How to Lose Everything: A Memoir.*

My friend **Leslie Davidson**, author of *Dancing in Small Spaces: One Couple's Journey With Parkinson's Disease and Lewy*

*Body Dementia,* has been so gracious in sharing her insight into the nature of suffering. **Ken Dalgleish** is also a friend and accomplished pianist. He has navigated several decades with multiple sclerosis and is always incredibly generous in shining his bright light on difficult-to-talk-about topics.

**Michael Klein** is yet another person we are lucky enough to call a friend. His work to address suffering is detailed in his book *Dissident Doctor: Catching Babies and Challenging the Medical Status Quo.* Michael has also experienced decades of painful neuropathy and brought an interesting dual outlook as both practitioner and pain sufferer.

**Kaliyana Denham-Rohlicek** is a young ballet dancer recently diagnosed with scoliosis that has caused an acute curvature in her spine. A gifted performer, Kaliyana relies heavily on a movement practice to find respite from the pain that accompanies her—like an unwanted chaperone—throughout her day.

And **John Alderson**, who spoke with me about his life after aggressive cancer treatment. We maintained an email conversation as I worked through a first, second, then third draft of this book. In the final days of 2020, Simon's cousin Lia called to relay the news that John had died. "A terrible end to a terrible year," she said. I am intensely grateful for the dialogue John and I shared during the final months of his life and offer my deepest sympathies to his wife, Val, and his two children.

It was not initially deliberate, but I came to see that I was seeking out people for whom, as Christa pointed out, "all better" was not an option. These were the stories I was hungry to hear: the difficulties, the strategies, and the unusual insight of people who grapple with the ongoing consequences of an illness, injury, or disorder. I wanted to know how it impacted their daily life and how it altered their vision for the future.

Each of these people, independently, thanked me for listening to their stories. Like Simon, they all were conscious of how uncomfortable their pain could make others feel. But it is I who is deeply indebted. Each of their unique perspectives expanded my understanding of this strange thing called pain, and their hard-won wisdom is threaded throughout these pages.

DEEP THANKS TO THE MANY PROFESSIONALS INTERVIEWED: Les Aria, Raju Heran, Nanna Brix Finnerup, Julian Taylor, Olaf Blanke, Paul Blakey, Jordan Kerton, Geordie Harrower, Lorimer Moseley, Joletta Belton, Tor Wager, Hance Clarke, Maria Hudspith, Michael Negraeff, Joerg Jaschinski, Rhonda Wilms, and Val Montessori. I was overwhelmed, often, by how generously they shared their time and expertise.

Other professionals also helped to direct and shape the book-writing process. Thank you Cathryn Jakobson Ramin, Neil Pearson, Devrit Srivastava, Eddie Berinstein, Daniel Goldberg, Howard Brody, Bernie Garrett, Jessica Archibald, Lynn Solomon, and John Kramer.

Thanks to our beloved friends and family who make cameos: Jay Johnson (who read an early draft and suggested the title), Boyd Norman, Paul Rigby, Walter Martella—aka Farm Team—you help fill our lives with music; Avi Lewis, who also brings music and passionate politics; Lia Paradis, Emily Paradis, Alice Paradis, Rachel Rose, Rob Stanley, Guido Heistek, Marc Paradis, and Lorna Paradis—all of whom did the thankless work of reading multiple drafts and providing constructive feedback. Thanks to our family at large, but specifically Eli and Emma—you are our everything.

The Sunshine Coast—trees, ocean, chattering ravens—is *home* to me. I am deeply grateful to live here, on the ancestral lands and unceded territory of the Coast Salish peoples—shíshálh (Sechelt), Sḵwx̱wú7mesh (Squamish), Stó:lō and Səl̓ílwətaʔ/Selilwitulh (Tsleil-Waututh) and xʷməθkʷəy̓əm (Musqueam) Nations. Chico, and our daily hikes, kept me sane during the book-writing process, as did the many conversations shared with my literary sisters: Jane Davidson, Amy Bespflug, Isabelle Denham, and Naomi and Bonnie Klein.

This project was completed with the support of both the Canada Council for the Arts through the Explore and Create grant program, and the BC Arts Council. The concept originated during a monthlong residency at the Banff Centre for Arts and Creativity in 2019, and I am forever grateful for that gift of time, encouragement, and guidance. Special thanks to Susan Orlean, Carol Shaben, Michael Harris, Jared Bland, and Kenneth Rosen. Andreas Schroeder and Sharon Oddie Brown provided a room-of-my-own in the form of an oceanside cabin, a gift beyond measure. Words cannot express my love and gratitude.

Thanks to my agent, Martha Webb, and to Greystone Books, who, in this era of solution-based books, took a leap on a project exploring uncertainty, contradiction, and pain. Special thanks to my vigilant editors, Nancy Flight and Paula Ayer, both of whom refused to let me settle.

And Simon. Thanks for agreeing—as you did so long ago—to go on this crazy journey with me.

# Notes

INTRODUCTION

2 **1.5 billion people:** D. S. Goldberg and S. J. McGee, "Pain as a Global Health Priority," *BMC Public Health* 11, no. 1 (Oct. 2011): 770.

2 **low back pain . . . has consistently been ranked as the number-one health care issue:** The WHO calculates the global burden of disease in YLDs, or "years lived with disability," and for more than two decades low back pain has been the top cause. Institute for Health Metrics and Evaluation (IHME), *Findings From the Global Burden of Disease Study 2017* (Seattle, WA: IHME, 2018), 13; A. Wu et al., "Global Low Back Prevalence and Years Lived With Disability From 1990 to 2017: Estimates From the Global Burden of Disease Study 2017," *Annals of Translational Medicine* 8, no. 6 (Mar. 2020): 299.

3 **In Canada, the estimated costs of chronic pain are roughly $60 billion:** Canadian Pain Task Force, *Chronic Pain in Canada: Laying a Foundation for Action*, June 2019, 11.

3 **In the U.S., that number is estimated to be somewhere between $560 and $635 billion:** D. J. Gaskin and P. Richard, "The Economic Costs of Pain in the United States," *Journal of Pain* 13, no. 8 (Aug. 2012), 715–24; CDC, "Health and Economic Costs of Chronic Diseases," cdc.gov/chronicdisease/about/costs/index.htm; National Cancer Institute, "Financial Burden of Cancer Care," April 2022, progressreport.cancer.gov/after/economic_burden.

I. AN ANNIVERSARY

11 **Eventually those journals and the accompanying research became a book:** *Fallen: A Trauma, a Marriage, and the Transformative Power of Music* was published in 2015 by Greystone Books. It tells the story of Simon's accident and his subsequent healing over the following five years.

15 **What do you do when acute pain strikes?:** Patrick Wall outlines these typical responses to acute pain in *Pain: The Science of Suffering* (New York: Columbia University Press, 2000, p. 150), noting that if any of these steps are frustrated, the associated pain postures and sensations may remain long after they are useful to the healing process.

16 **I turned to scientific journals, reading everything I could about pain after spinal cord injury:** D. Burke et al., "Neuropathic Pain Prevalence Following

Spinal Cord Injury: A Systemic Review and Meta-Analysis," *European Journal of Pain* 21, no. 1 (Jan. 2017): 29–44; S. D. Guy et al., "The CanPain SCI Clinical Practice Guidelines for Rehabilitation Management of Neuropathic Pain After Spinal Cord: Recommendations for Treatment," *Spinal Cord* 54, suppl. 1 (Aug. 2016): S14–23.

## 2. INTRODUCING RUPERT

26 **"The relief of pain is obviously one of the main functions of physicians," psychiatrist Frank Ervin said:** "Attack on Pain," *Time,* Mar. 2, 1959. Quoted in Keith Wailoo's excellent book *Pain: A Political History* (Baltimore: Johns Hopkins University Press, 2014), 30.

26 **a review of pain education:** Canadian Pain Task Force, *Chronic Pain in Canada*, 21.

26 **Internationally the picture is no better:** E. E. Shipton et al., "Systematic Review of Pain Medicine Content, Teaching, and Assessment in Medical School Curricula Internationally," *Pain Therapy* 7, no. 2 (Dec. 2018): 139–61.

27 **pain as a "need state" that, like hunger or thirst:** Wall, *Pain*, 152.

27 **One of my favorite chapters . . . characterizes pain as an odious bore:** Marni Jackson, *Pain: The Fifth Vital Sign* (New York: Crown, 2002), 97. Within a brilliant, informative, and charming book this chapter ("Pain as a Bore," 95–99) is a standout. It is *the* most accurate and wittily rendered account of bodily pain I read over the course of my research.

32 **most commonly imagined as "gates":** The "gate control theory" of pain was pioneered by Ronald Melzack and Patrick Wall and outlined in their paradigm-shifting publication *The Challenge of Pain: Exciting Discoveries in the New Science of Pain Control* (New York: Basic Books, 1983).

34 **a conversation between his central and peripheral nervous system:** The nervous system regulates all functions of the body—breathing, digestion, voluntary movement, consciousness—and is structurally divided into two main parts: the central nervous system (CNS) and the peripheral nervous system (PNS). The CNS comprises the brain, brain stem, and spinal cord; the PNS is made up of all the peripheral nerves that branch out from the spinal cord, enervating the limbs and organs.

35 **Pain, we also learned, always has a context:** "To effectively deal with pain, it is important to identify the contextual cues. We like to call them the cues that help ignite a pain experience, or 'ignition cues.'" G. Lorimer Moseley and David Butler, *Explain Pain* (Adelaide, Australia: Noigroup, 2013), 18–21.

35 **Various studies:** Moseley and Butler, *Explain Pain,* 17–21; Wall, *Pain,* 133.

36 **men wounded in battle:** Melzack and Wall, *Challenge of Pain*, 35. Henry Beecher's seminal research is oft cited as a demonstration of how powerfully contextual factors can influence the in-the-moment experience of pain.

38 **Pain and tissue damage are related, but they are not the same thing:** Moseley and Butler, *Explain Pain,* 12.

38 **the complicated relationship between tissue damage and perceived pain:** G. Lorimer Moseley's TEDx Talk "Why Things Hurt" (Nov. 21, 2011) is also

a dramatic illustration of this point. He is a fabulous storyteller who makes key tenets of pain science both accessible and entertaining: youtube.com/watch?v=gwd-wLd1Hjs.

38 **A twenty-nine-year-old British construction worker:** J. P. Fisher, D. T. Hassan, and N. O'Connor, Minerva (column), *British Medical Journal* 310 (Jan. 1995): 70; M. Johnson, "Trauma and Pain: A Fragile Link," *Journal of Trauma and Treatment* 6, no. 2 (May 2017).

40 **neuroscientist V. S. Ramachandran:** V. S. Ramachandran, *The Tell-Tale Brain: A Neuroscientist's Quest for What Makes Us Human* (New York: W. W. Norton, 2012), 33.

3. AN ACTION PLAN

51 **Ronald Melzack... challenged this perspective:** R. Melzack, "From the Gate to the Neuromatrix," *Pain* 6, suppl. (Aug. 1999): S121–26.

51 ***allostatic load*:** B. McEwan, "Stressed or Stressed Out: What Is the Difference?" *Journal of Psychiatry and Neuroscience* 30, no. 5 (Sept. 2005): 315–18; M. K. Nicholas, "Why Do Some People Develop Chronic, Treatment-Resistant Pain and Not Others?" *Pain* 159, no. 12 (Dec. 2018): 2419–20; D. Borsook et al., "When Pain Gets Stuck: The Evolution of Pain Chronification and Treatment Resistance," *Pain* 159, no. 12 (Dec. 2018): 2421–36.

52 **It's not unusual for anxiety, stress, and pain states to be intimately connected:** G. J. G. Asmundson et al., "PTSD and the Experience of Pain: Research and Clinical Implications of Shared Vulnerability and Mutual Maintenance Models," *Canadian Journal of Psychiatry* 47, no. 10 (Dec. 2002): 930–36; G. J. G. Asmundson and J. Katz, "Understanding the Co-Occurrence of Anxiety Disorder and Chronic Pain: State-of-the-Art," *Depression and Anxiety* 26, no. 10 (Oct. 2009): 888–901; R. Defrin, Y. Lahav, and Z. Solomon, "Dysfunctional Pain Modulation in Torture Survivors: The Mediating Effect of PTSD," *Journal of Pain* 18, no. 1 (Jan. 2017): 1–10.

54 **thinking inside and outside of the box: Feldenkrais** refers to the awareness-through-movement strategies developed by the iconic Moshé Feldenkrais. **Craniosacral therapy** is a gentle, hands-on technique developed by osteopathic physician John E. Upledger. Using a light touch, a CST therapist explores the movement of fluids in and around the central nervous system with the aim of releasing tension deep in the body. **Intramuscular stimulation** is also referred to as "dry needling." Physiotherapists use very fine needles—like those used in acupuncture—to release or lengthen muscles that may be contributing to chronic musculoskeletal or neuropathic pain. A Vancouver-based physician, Chan Gunn, developed IMS in the 1970s and currently offers certification to medical professionals at his Institute for the Study and Treatment of Pain at the University of British Columbia. **Nerve blocks** work by injecting medication into specific clusters of nerves. Many types of nerve blocks are available to address different types of pain, and they are used for a variety of therapeutic purposes. **TENS (transcutaneous electrical nerve stimulation) machines**

are small battery-operated devices developed by the pain-research maverick Patrick Wall. The device is attached to the skin by sticky patches connected to electrodes that deliver small electrical pulses to the body. While there is little data to support the use of TENS, many people find them extremely helpful. In theory, the steady electrical impulse is meant to distract and reduce pain-provoking signals from traveling to the spinal cord and brain, helping to reduce overall pain and relax muscles. TENS is noninvasive and generally risk free.

56 **John Bonica:** Bonica imagined clinics that offered a constellation of therapeutic interventions from a range of professionals: anesthesiologists, nurses, physical and occupational therapists, neurologists, surgeons, psychologists, pharmacists, dieticians, and social workers. Depending on the patient's needs, these professionals would coordinate to create a comprehensive treatment plan. Research highlights that, in contrast to isolated interventions like surgery or medication, an integrated approach is more effective in limiting pain distress and disability. Patients of multidisciplinary programs have improved physical functioning, faster return to work, and are less likely to require further medical interventions. Marcia Meldrum, "Brief History of Multidisciplinary Management of Chronic Pain, 1900–2000," in *Chronic Pain Management: Guidelines for Multidisciplinary Program Development*, ed. M. E. Schatman and A. Campbell (New York: Informa, 2007), 6–7; U. Kaiser, R.-D. Treede, and R. Sabatowski, "Multimodal Pain Therapy in Chronic Noncancer Pain—Gold Standard or Need for Further Clarification?" *Pain* 158, no. 10 (Oct. 2017): 1853–59; R. D. Kerns, E. E. Krebs, and D. Atkins, "Making Integrated Multimodal Pain Care a Reality: A Path Forward," *Journal of General Internal Medicine* 33, suppl. 1 (May 2018): 1–3; J. G. Pilitsis, O. Khazen, and N. G. Wenzel, "Multidisciplinary Firms and the Treatment of Chronic Pain: A Case Study of Low Back Pain," *Frontiers in Pain Research* 2 (Nov. 2021); Canadian Pain Task Force, *Chronic Pain in Canada.*

56 **still not a widely available option:** M. Choinière et al., "Accessing Care in Multidisciplinary Pain Treatment Facilities Continues to Be a Challenge in Canada," *Regional Anesthesia and Pain Medicine* 45, no. 12 (Dec. 2020): 943–48.

## 4. PSYKHĒ SŌMATIKOS

61 **more detail-oriented questionnaires do exist:** The basic test most of us are familiar with is the **Numerical Rating Scale (NRS)**, an 11-point scale where 0 = no pain and 10 = the worst pain imaginable. The **Visual Analogue Scale (VAS)** is a variant of the NRS. The **Verbal Rating Scale (VRS)**, another variant, uses words—none, mild, moderate, severe—to describe the magnitude of a person's pain. Chronic pain, ideally, requires a more detailed questionnaire. Ron Melzack created the **McGill Pain Questionnaire**, which uses a series of descriptive words to assess a patient's sensory, cognitive, and evaluative experience of pain. Widely used in research, it's deemed highly reliable in assessing both acute and chronic pain states. The **Brief Pain Inventory (BPI)** uses a numerical rating scale to measure 1) pain intensity; 2) pain relief from current treatment;

3) pain's interference in a person's daily life. The **LANSS Pain Scale**, **DN4**, **PainDETECT**, and **Neuropathic Pain Scale** are all used to determine if pain has the complication of being neuropathic. Further questionnaires investigate levels of anxiety, depression, tendency to catastrophize pain, or confidence in self-management. Others assess pain in children or nonverbal patients. The article cited below offers a comprehensive listing of all pain rating scales in current use.

I tend to agree with Simon that assigning a numerical value to chronic pain is an imperfect attempt at assessing someone's state of being. The real value of these questionnaires is in their ability to track short- and long-term patterns. Knowing which assessment tools are available is also useful in self-advocacy. If you're having a difficult time communicating with a health care provider and feel that certain facets of your pain experience are being consistently overlooked, suggesting one of these questionnaires might provide a bridge to a more productive conversation. See T. Bendinger and N. Plunkett, "Measurement in Pain Medicine," *BJA Education* 16, no. 9 (Sept. 2016): 310–15.

68 **This was true even for Descartes:** Joanna Bourke, *The Story of Pain: From Prayer to Painkillers* (Oxford: Oxford University Press, 2014), 241; René Descartes, "Meditations on First Philosophy," trans. Elizabeth S. Haldane and G. R. T. Ross, in *Descartes: Key Philosophical Writings,* ed. Enrique Chávez-Arizo and Tom Griffith (Ware, UK: Wordsworth, 1997), 183.

69 **medical historian Roy Porter:** R. Porter, "Oh, My Aching Back," *London Review of Books* 17, no. 21 (Nov. 1995).

70 **Elaine Scarry:** Elaine Scarry, *The Body in Pain* (New York: Oxford University Press, 1985), 7.

## 5. WELCOMING THE UNWELCOME

75 **"normal abnormalities":** Issues discovered on scans do not always correlate with the experience of felt pain. In 1990, orthopedic surgeon Scott Bogden ran scans on sixty-seven people without back pain. The results were shocking: 90 percent had degenerated or bulging discs, while 33 percent had herniated discs. A Mayo Clinic study demonstrated that disc degeneration was present for asymptomatic people of all ages. Subjects in their twenties had a more than 33 percent chance of having disc anomalies; over forty, roughly 50 percent; over sixty, a whopping 90 percent. But all these test subjects were pain-free. Cathryn J. Ramin, *Crooked: Outwitting the Back Pain Industry and Getting on the Road to Recovery* (New York: HarperCollins, 2017), 46, 52–53.

75 **tension myositis syndrome:** TMS is also referred to as tension myoneural syndrome or MindBody syndrome.

80 **Created by Stephen Porges, the Safe and Sound Protocol:** The Polyvagal Institute has a comprehensive list of Porges's research articles at polyvagalinstitute .org/authored-by-dr-porges.

82 **acceptance and commitment therapy:** Joanne Dahl and Tobias Lundgren, "Acceptance and Commitment Therapy (ACT) in the Treatment of Chronic

Pain," in *Mindfulness-Based Treatment Approaches: Clinician's Guide to Evidence Base and Applications*, ed. R. A. Baer (London: Elsevier, 2006), 285–306.

84 **researchers at Indiana University:** The Kinsey Institute is home to the Traumatic Stress Research Consortium: polyvagalinstitute.org/kinsey.

84 **Unyte:** The Unyte support team was helpful and provided ongoing access to educational resources: unyte.com.

85 **an unapologetic mindfulness propaganda campaign:** Moshé Feldenkrais, *Awareness Through Movement* (New York: HarperCollins, 1990); Jon Kabat-Zinn, *Full Catastrophe Living: Using the Wisdom of Your Body and Mind to Face Stress, Pain, and Illness* (New York: Bantam, 2013); H. Kober et al., "Let It Be: Mindful Acceptance Down-Regulates Pain and Negative Emotion," *Social Cognitive and Affective Neuroscience* 14, no. 11 (Nov. 2019): 1147–58; A. Doll et al., "Mindful Attention to Breath Regulates Emotions via Increased Amygdala-Prefrontal Cortex Connectivity," *NeuroImage* 134 (2016): 305–13; E.-L. Khoo et al., "Comparative Evaluation of Group-Based Mindfulness-Based Stress Reduction and Cognitive Behavioral Therapy for the Treatment and Management of Chronic Pain: A Systematic Review and Network Meta-Analysis," *Evidence Based Mental Health* 22, no. 1 (Feb. 2019): 26–35.

## 6. A DOG WITH CHOICES

93 **Studies conducted both at the Adelaide Medical School by Mark Hutchinson and at the University of Texas by Peter Grace:** M. R. Hutchinson et al., "Exploring the Neuroimmunopharmacology of Opioids: An Integrative Review of Mechanisms of Central Immune Signaling and Their Implications for Opioid Analgesia," *Pharmacological Reviews* 63, no. 3 (Sept. 2011): 772–810; S. M. Green-Fulgham et al., "Oxycodone, Fentanyl, and Morphine Amplify Established Neuropathic Pain in Male Rats," *Pain* 160, no. 11 (Nov. 2019): 2634–40; G. Lorimer Moseley and David Butler, *Explain Pain Supercharged* (Adelaide, Australia: Noigroup, 2017), 59.

## 7. GROOVES AND RUTS

103 **the brain as a brilliant cartographer:** Antonio Damasio, *Self Comes to Mind: Constructing the Conscious Brain* (New York: Pantheon, 2010), 64. "The human brain is a born cartographer, and the cartography began with the mapping of the body inside which the brain sits."

104 **intense musical training promotes neuroplasticity:** C. Y. Wan and G. Schlaug, "Music Making as a Tool for Promoting Brain Plasticity Across the Life Span," *Neuroscientist* 16, no. 5 (Oct. 2010): 566–77.

## 8. THE EXPECTATION EFFECT

116 **Patrick Wall and Ron Melzack believed:** Melzack and Wall, *Challenge of Pain*, 84–86, 297.

118 **The negative connotations of the word *placebo*:** A. J. de Crean et al., "Placebos and Placebo Effects in Medicine: Historical Overview," *Journal of the Royal*

*Society of Medicine* 92, no. 10 (Oct. 1999): 511–15; John Haygarth, *Of the Imagination, as a Cause and as a Cure of Disorders of the Body; Exemplified by Fictitious Tractors, and Epidemical Convulsions* (Bath: R. Cruttwell, 1800).

120 **"unintelligent, neurotic, or inadequate patients":** de Crean et al., "Placebos and Placebo Effects," 511; R. P. C. Handfield-Jones, "A Bottle of Medicine From the Doctor," *Lancet* 262, no. 6790 (Oct. 1953): 823–25.

120 **"graveyard of drug discovery":** "'Be Ambitious. Go for the Big Questions': A Conversation With Irene Tracey." This interview was part of a podcast series created for the North American Pain School in 2018. It's also where I first heard Dr. Tracey's pitch to rename the *placebo effect* as the *expectation effect.*

120 **a study performed at Eastman Dental Hospital:** Wall, *Pain*, 127–28.

121 **Some of the latest research:** I. Tracey, "Finding the Hurt in Pain," *Cerebrum* (Dec. 2016).

122 **the expectation effect is active even in a surgical context:** K. Wartolowska et al., "Use of Placebo Controls in the Evaluation of Surgery: Systematic Review," *British Medical Journal* 348 (May 2014): g3253; K. Wartolowska et al., "A Meta-Analysis of Temporal Changes of Response in the Placebo Arm of Surgical Randomized Controlled Trials: An Update," *Trials* 18, article no. 323 (July 2017).

9. THE KING OF FAKE NEWS

129 ***Neuroplastic Transformation* workbook:** Michael Moskowitz and Marla Golden, *Neuroplastic Transformation: Your Brain on Pain* (Neuroplastic Partners, 2013), 6–7.

134 **The workbook advises looking at the pain-free graphic:** Moskowitz and Golden, *Neuroplastic Transformation,* 12.

134 ***The Brain's Way of Healing*:** Norman Doidge, "Physician Hurt, Then Heal Thyself: Michael Moskowitz Discovers That Chronic Pain Can Be Unlearned," in *The Brain's Way of Healing: Remarkable Discoveries and Recoveries From the Frontiers of Neuroplasticity* (New York: Penguin, 2016), 1–32.

134 **the scent of peppermint helps block substance P:** Moskowitz and Golden, *Neuroplastic Transformation,* 47–48.

135 **the tenth cranial, or vagus, nerve:** Moskowitz and Golden, *Neuroplastic Transformation,* 68.

136 **GABA:** gamma-aminobutyric acid is a neurotransmitter released during soothing activities that helps prevent inflammation and promote activity in the pleasure circuits of the brain.

11. BE EASY, BRUV

161 **the same minor finger injury:** G. Lorimer Moseley and David Butler, *The Explain Pain Handbook: Protectometer* (Adelaide, Australia: Noigroup, 2015), 11; Moseley and Butler, *Explain Pain,* 18.

161 ***biopsychosocial* experience:** Moseley and Butler, *Explain Pain Supercharged,* 12–14; G. L. Engel, "The Need for a New Medical Model: A Challenge for

Biomedicine," *Science* 196, no. 4286 (Apr. 1977): 129–36; F. Borrell-Carrió, A. L. Suchman, and R. M. Epstein, "The Biopsychosocial Model 25 Years Later: Principles, Practice, and Scientific Inquiry," *Annals of Family Medicine* 2, no. 6 (Nov. 2004): 576–82.

161 **Their research demonstrates:** G. L. Moseley and D. S. Butler, "Fifteen Years of Explaining Pain: The Past, Present and Future," *Journal of Pain* 16, no. 9 (June 2015): 807–13; G. L. Moseley, "Unravelling the Barriers to Reconceptualization of the Problem in Chronic Pain: The Actual and Perceived Ability of Patients and Health Professionals to Understand the Neurophysiology," *Journal of Pain* 4, no. 4 (May 2003): 184–89; G. L. Moseley, "Combined Physiotherapy and Education Is Efficacious for Chronic Low Back Pain," *Australian Journal of Physiotherapy* 48, no. 4 (2002): 297–302.

161 **identify their DIMS:** Moseley and Butler, *Protectometer*, 14–27.

162 **Expanding *neuroplastic* to *bioplastic*:** Moseley and Butler, *Protectometer*, 30.

162 **"We believe that all pain experiences are normal":** Moseley and Butler, *Explain Pain*, 8.

167 ***shinrin-yoku*:** M. M. Hansen, R. Jones, and K. Tocchini, "Shinrin-Yoku (Forest Bathing) and Nature Therapy: A State-of-the-Art Review," *International Journal of Environmental Research and Public Health* 14, no. 8 (July 2017): 851; "What the Heck Is Forest Bathing? 5 Things You Didn't Know About Shinrin-Yoku in BC," Super, Natural British Columbia, April 2017, hellobc.com/stories/what-the-heck-is-forest-bathing-5-things-you-didnt-know-about-shinrin-yoku-in-bc.

### 13. INSIDER INFO

190 **"the North American opioid crisis":** L. Degenhardt et al., "Global Patterns of Opioid Use and Dependence: Harms to Populations, Interventions, and Future Action," *Lancet* 394, no. 10208 (Oct. 2019): 1560–79. "In high income countries, increased prescribing of opioids for chronic non-cancer pain has produced iatrogenic dependence and subsequent increase in illicit opioid use, most prominently in the USA and Canada." See also Wailoo, *Pain*, 191; L. Manchikanti and A. Singh, "Therapeutic Opioids: A Ten-Year Perspective on the Complexities and Complications of the Escalating Use, Abuse, and Nonmedical Use of Opioids," *Pain Physician* 11 (Opioid Special Issue, 2008): 563–88; United Nations Office on Drugs and Crime, *World Drug Report 2021*, 18, 46, unodc.org/unodc/en/data-and-analysis/wdr2021.html.

193 **"Garden Snails cleansed and bruised":** "Top Hospital and Medical Facts," Old Operating Theatre Museum and Herb Garret, oldoperatingtheatre.com/top-hospital-medical-facts.

193 **Novelist Fanny Burney provides a detailed account:** Fanny Burney titled the letter "Account From Paris of a Terrible Operation." The full transcript is available at the British Library website, part of the Berg Collection, New York Public Library: bl.uk/collection-items/letter-from-frances-burney-to-her-sister-esther-about-her-mastectomy.

## 14. TIME IS ART

205 **"principles presented in this book":** Moseley and Butler, *Explain Pain*, 5.

210 **one paper specific to VR interventions for people with spinal cord injuries:** P. Pozeg et al., "Virtual Reality Improves Embodiment and Neuropathic Pain Caused by Spinal Cord Injury," *Neurology* 89, no. 18 (Oct. 2017): 1894–1903. I have since discovered another article: M. Solcà et al., "Enhancing Analgesic Spinal Cord Stimulation for Chronic Pain With Personalized Immersive Virtual Reality," *Pain* 162, no. 6 (June 2021): 1641–49; as well, an earlier, small-scale study authored by G. Lorimer Moseley, while not explicitly using VR technology, has implications for its potential success: G. L. Moseley, "Using Visual Illusion to Reduce At-Level Neuropathic Pain in Paraplegia," *Pain* 130, no. 3 (Aug. 2007): 294–98.

212 **"Visualizing a line of movement through the body":** Irene Dowd, *Taking Root to Fly: Articles on Functional Anatomy* (self-pub., 1995), 2.

212 **In 1995, Alvaro Pascual-Leone:** A. Pascual-Leone et al., "Modulation of Muscle Responses Evoked by Transcranial Magnetic Stimulation During the Acquisition of New Fine Motor Skills," *Journal of Neurophysiology* 74, no. 3 (Sept. 1995): 1037–45.

## 15. THE MEANING OF PAIN

219 **International medical science, so far, does not wholly agree:** S. Haroutounian et al., "International Association for the Study of Pain Presidential Task Force on Cannabis and Cannabinoid Analgesia: Research Agenda on the Use of Cannabinoids, Cannabis, and Cannabis-Based Medicines for Pain Management," *Pain* 162, suppl. 1 (July 2021): S117–24; M. Mohiuddin et al., "General Risks of Harm With Cannabinoids, Cannabis, and Cannabis-Based Medicine Possibly Relevant to Patients Receiving These for Pain Management: An Overview of Systematic Reviews," *Pain* 162, suppl. 1 (July 2021): S80–96.

220 **David Morris argues:** David B. Morris, *The Culture of Pain* (Berkeley and Los Angeles, CA: University of California Press, 1991), 26, 29.

222 **"To suspend it by artificial agency":** Skey, "Result of the Use of Chloroform in 9000 Cases at Bartholomew's Hospital," *Buffalo Medical Journal and Monthly Review of Medical and Surgical Science* 7 (1851–52): 108, cited in Bourke, *Story of Pain*, 279.

222 **James Young Simpson pioneered the use of chloroform:** Bourke, *Story of Pain*, 283–84.

222 **"Chloroform... was a decoy of Satan":** Draft letter from James Young Simpson to Dr. Protheroe Smith (quoting an anonymous clergyman), 1848, Royal College of Surgeons of Edinburgh archives, JYS 232, quoted in Bourke, *Story of Pain*, 283.

222 **"caustic old maids":** Draft letter from James Young Simpson, quoted in Bourke, *Story of Pain*, 284.

223 **"Even the slightest sensory disturbances":** René Leriche, *The Surgery of Pain*, trans. Archibald Young (London: Ballière, Tindall and Co., 1938), 56–57, quoted in Bourke, *Story of Pain*, 200.

16. U-DREAM

233 **Mrs. Winslow's Soothing Syrup:** Sam Quinones, *Dreamland: The True Tale of America's Opiate Epidemic* (New York: Bloomsbury, 2015), 53.

234 **Harrison Narcotics Tax Act:** Quinones, *Dreamland*, 54.

234 **The claims Purdue made weren't true:** Quinones, *Dreamland*, 264–69.

234 **a Purdue-funded study of headache sufferers:** Patrick Radden Keefe, "The Family That Built an Empire of Pain," *New Yorker*, Oct. 23, 2017.

235 **in 1997 there were 670,000 oxy prescriptions for chronic pain . . . in 2002, that number rose to 6.2 million:** Quinones, *Dreamland*, 138.

235 **exploit the divisive nature of American politics:** This is a position convincingly argued in Wailoo, *Pain*, 169.

236 **overdoses in numbers that exceeded deaths due to car crashes:** Quinones, *Dreamland*, 203, 249. Quinones describes how, in 2007, epidemiologist Ed Socie and his supervisor, Christy Beeghly, dissected the shocking incoming data on drug overdoses in Ohio, realizing that "drug overdose deaths were about to surpass fatal auto crashes as Ohio's top cause of injury death. This," Quinones writes, "was a stunning moment in the history of U.S. public health . . . Drug overdoses passed fatal vehicle accidents nationwide for the first time in 2008."

236 **approximately 564,000 overdose deaths from opioids:** Wide-Ranging Online Data for Epidemiologic Research (WONDER), CDC, National Center for Health Statistics, 2020, wonder.cdc.gov. A May 11, 2022, CDC update indicates that there were over eighty thousand overdose deaths involving opioids in the U.S. in 2021: cdc.gov/nchs/pressroom/nchs_press_releases/2022/202205.htm.

236 **Silas Weir Mitchell had warned:** Bourke, *Story of Pain*, 281.

237 **multiple class-action lawsuits:** In October 2020, Purdue pled guilty to federal criminal charges and was fined $8 billion. In 2023, the Sackler family, who owns Purdue Pharma, agreed to a bankruptcy plan that required them personally to place an additional $6 billion into a trust fund used to pay out further claims against the company. In exchange, the Sacklers will be shielded from any ongoing consequences of litigation. In 2020, unprecedented charges were laid against executives at Insys Therapeutics, a company that followed in the footsteps of Purdue in their aggressive marketing of the even more powerful drug fentanyl. Charged under the Racketeer Influenced and Corrupt Organizations (RICO) Act, Insys executives will join the ranks of mob bosses and drug lords, the trial sending an important message that drug company executives will be held criminally accountable for their actions in the future. Dietrich Knauth, "Purdue Pharma Can Protect Sackler Owners in Opioid Bankruptcy," Reuters, May 30, 2023, reuters.com/legal/purdue-pharma-can-protect-sackler-owners-opioid-bankruptcy-court-rules-2023-05-30; Peter J. Henning, "RICO Offers a Powerful Tool to Punish Executives for the Opioid Crisis," *New York Times*, May 23, 2019; U. S. Attorney's Office, District of Massachusetts, "Founder and Four Executives of Insys Therapeutics

Convicted of Racketeering Conspiracy," press release, May 2, 2019, justice.gov/usao-ma/pr/founder-and-four-executives-insys-therapeutics-convicted-racketeering-conspiracy.

238 **"recalled U-Dream":** At the time of writing, U-Dream is not available in Canada.

17. STEP FIVE

242 **Joletta Belton:** Joletta Belton, *My Cuppa Jo* (blog), mycuppajo.substack.com.

247 **the Cognitive and Affective Neuroscience Lab at Dartmouth College:** sites.dartmouth.edu/canlab.

248 **a paper published in the *New England Journal of Medicine*:** T. Wager et al., "An fMRI-Based Neurologic Signature of Physical Pain," *New England Journal of Medicine* 368 (Apr. 2013): 1388–97.

253 **Transitional Pain Service:** transitionalpainservice.ca.

255 **Medical Cannabis Real-World Evidence:** mcrwe.ca. In 2021, Hance Clarke, along with nineteen other experts from nine countries, made recommendations on dosing and administering medical cannabis for people with chronic pain. A. Bhaskar et al., "Consensus Recommendation of Medical Cannabis to Treat Chronic Pain: Results of a Modified Delphi Process," *Journal of Cannabis Research* 3, no. 1 (July 2021): 22.

19. A QUESTION AS YET UNANSWERED

266 **our metaphoric language matters:** Four great references for thinking about how our figurative language helps to define and create the experience of pain are Moseley and Butler, "The Malleable Magic of Metaphor," chap. 7 in *Explain Pain Supercharged*, 143–68; S. Neilson, "Pain as Metaphor: Metaphor and Medicine," *Medical Humanities* 42, no. 1 (Mar. 2016): 3–10; Bourke, chap. 3 in *The Story of Pain*, 53–87; George Lakoff, "The Neural Theory of Metaphor," chap. 1 in *The Cambridge Handbook of Metaphor and Thought*, ed. Raymond W. Gibbs, Jr. (Cambridge: Cambridge University Press, 2008), 17–38, available at escholarship.org/content/qt9n6745m6/qt9n6745m6_noSplash_a28b21eb20fc0a67c0d7600f9205525e.pdf.

268 **pain . . . is viewed as too complex:** M. Cohen, J. Quintner, and D. Buchanan, "Is Chronic Pain a Disease?" *Pain Medicine* 14, no. 9 (Sept. 2013): 1284–88.

277 **Michael created his own blog space:** Michael Negraeff, *Narratives From the Neuromatrix: Where Science and Humanity Meet* (blog), michaelnegraeff.com.

278 **"The meaning of pain":** Morris, *Culture of Pain*, 26.

20. ANOTHER ANNIVERSARY

280 **The Leap Manifesto:** leapmanifesto.org.

281 **a short film collaboration with the artist Molly Crabapple:** "A Message From the Future With Alexandria Ocasio-Cortez," The Intercept, Apr. 17, 2019, video, 7:35, theintercept.com/2019/04/17/green-new-deal-short-film-alexandria-ocasio-cortez/.

281 **statistics from the Oxfam website:** Oxfam International, "Not All Gaps Are Created Equal: The True Value of Care Work," oxfam.org/en/not-all-gaps-are-created-equal-true-value-care-work. This is an excellent resource in parsing out the economic implications of unpaid care work.

282 **an image used by... Jeffrey Rediger:** Jeffrey Rediger, *Cured: Strengthen Your Immune System and Heal Your Life* (New York: Flatiron, 2020), 40.

283 **"Denmark's a good practical example":** See André Picard, *Neglected No More: The Urgent Need to Improve the Lives of Canada's Elders in the Wake of a Pandemic* (Toronto: Random House Canada, 2021), 146.

### 22. THE THING WITH FEATHERS

309 **More people in British Columbia died of overdose:** British Columbia Government News, "B.C. Experiences Record Loss of Life Due to Drug Toxicity," news release, Dec. 9, 2021, news.gov.bc.ca/releases/2021PSSG0099-002356; BC Centre for Disease Control, "Knowledge Update," Sept. 15, 2021, bccdc.ca/resource-gallery/Documents/Statistics%20and%20Research/Statistics%20and%20Reports/Overdose/2021.09.15_Knowledge%20Update_Hydromorphone%20and%20drug%20toxicity%20deaths.pdf.

309 **"Since 2016 overdose deaths in B.C.":** Pain BC, "Addressing Chronic Pain and Overdose in the Trades," Jan. 15, 2021, painbc.ca/blog/addressing-chronic-pain-and-overdose-trades.

312 **"Hard Times":** "Hard Times," © 2011. Written by Gillian Welch and David Rawlings. Published by Acony Publishing (BMI) and 3rd Revision (BMI). Used with Permission. All rights reserved.

# Selected Bibliography

To understand pain as a biological, psychological, cultural, economic, and political problem required approaching the topic from many different angles. This core bibliography provided an excellent foundation.


Bourke, Joanna. *The Story of Pain: From Prayer to Painkillers.* Oxford: Oxford University Press, 2014.

Canadian Pain Task Force. *An Action Plan for Pain in Canada.* Ottawa, ON: Health Canada, 2021.

Canadian Pain Task Force. *Chronic Pain in Canada: Laying a Foundation for Action.* Ottawa, ON: Health Canada, 2019.

Canadian Pain Task Force. *Working Together to Better Understand, Prevent and Manage Chronic Pain: What We Heard.* Ottawa, ON: Health Canada, 2020. All three reports are available at canada.ca/en/health-canada/corporate/about-health-canada/public-engagement/external-advisory-bodies/canadian-pain-task-force/reports-meetings.html.

The Care Collective. *The Care Manifesto: The Politics of Interdependence.* London and New York: Verso, 2020.

Cassell, Eric J. *The Nature of Suffering and the Goals of Medicine.* New York: Oxford University Press, 1991.

Jackson, Marni. *Pain: The Fifth Vital Sign.* New York: Crown, 2002.

Jakobson Ramin, Cathryn. *Crooked: Outwitting the Back Pain Industry and Getting on the Road to Recovery.* New York: HarperCollins, 2017.

Melzack, Ronald, and Patrick Wall. *The Challenge of Pain: Exciting Discoveries in the New Science of Pain Control.* New York: Basic Books, 1983.

Morris, David B. *The Culture of Pain.* Berkeley and Los Angeles, California: University of California Press, 1991.

Moseley, G. Lorimer. *Painful Yarns: Metaphors and Stories to Help Understand the Biology of Pain.* Canberra, Australia: Dancing Giraffe, 2007.

Moseley, G. Lorimer, and David Butler. *Explain Pain.* Explain Pain series. Adelaide, Australia: Noigroup, 2013.

Moseley, G. Lorimer, and David Butler. *The Explain Pain Handbook: Protectometer.* Explain Pain series. Adelaide, Australia: Noigroup, 2015.

Moseley, G. Lorimer, and David Butler. *Explain Pain Supercharged.* Explain Pain series. Adelaide, Australia: Noigroup, 2017.

Moskowitz, Michael, and Marla Golden. *Neuroplastic Transformation: Your Brain on Pain.* Neuroplastic Partners, 2013.

Porges, Stephen W. *The Pocket Guide to the Polyvagal Theory: The Transformative Power of Feeling Safe.* New York: W. W. Norton, 2017.

Porges, Stephen W. *The Polyvagal Theory: Neurophysiological Foundations of Emotions, Attachment, Communication, and Self-Regulation.* New York: W. W. Norton, 2011.

Quinones, Sam. *Dreamland: The True Tale of America's Opiate Epidemic.* New York: Bloomsbury, 2015.

Wailoo, Keith. *Pain: A Political History.* Baltimore: John Hopkins University Press, 2014.

Wall, Patrick. *Pain: The Science of Suffering.* New York: Columbia University Press, 2000.

## ONLINE PAIN RESOURCE GUIDE

The Pain Resource Guide, available at **greystonebooks.com/products/the-pain-project**, offers further discussion of neuropathic pain, including a list of possible indicators that pain may be in part neuroplastic in nature. Critically important yet often maddeningly elusive, the health of the nervous system is difficult to address; this online resource provides some tips. Included is an exploration of the importance of a movement practice (in contrast to the more common idea of an exercise regime) along with an overview of the possible benefits, cautions, affordability, and accessibility of yoga, Pilates, Feldenkrais, qigong, tai chi, and Alexander Technique.